2003

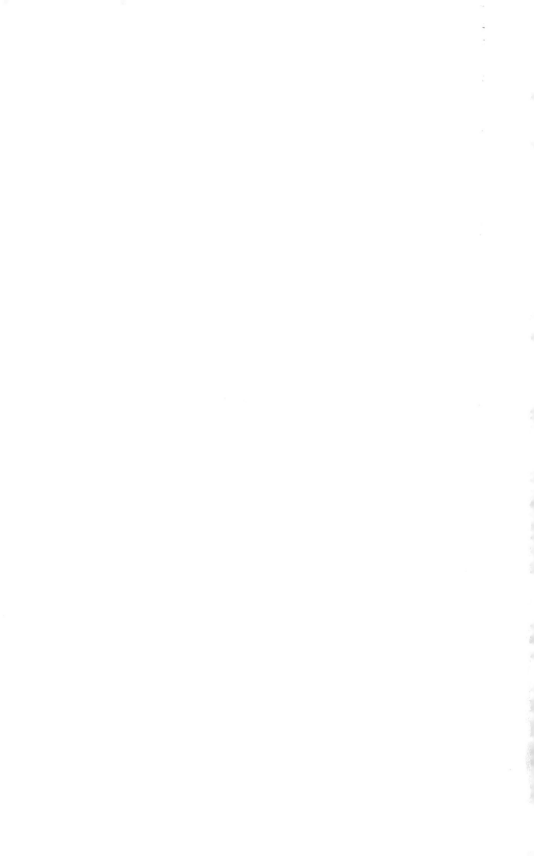

The Jossey-Bass Health Care Series brings together the most current information and ideas in health care from the leaders in the field. Titles from the Jossey-Bass Health Care Series include these essential health care resources:

Beyond Managed Care

Beyond Managed Care

How Consumers and Technology Are Changing the Future of Health Care

Dean C. Coddington, Elizabeth A. Fischer,

Keith D. Moore, Richard L. Clarke

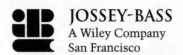

JOSSEY-BASS
A Wiley Company
San Francisco

Jossey-Bass books and products are available through most bookstores. To contact Jossey-Bass directly, call (888) 378-2537, fax to (800) 605-2665, or visit our website at www.josseybass.com.

Substantial discounts on bulk quantities of Jossey-Bass books are available to corporations, professional associations, and other organizations. For details and discount information, contact the special sales department at Jossey-Bass.

Credits are on page 335.

 Manufactured in the United States of America on Lyons Falls Turin Book. This paper is acid-free and 100 percent totally chlorine-free.

Library of Congress Cataloging-in-Publication Data
Beyond managed care : how consumers and technology are changing the future of health care / Dean Coddington . . . [et al.].
   p.   cm.
Includes bibliographical references and index.
   ISBN 0-7879-5383-0
   1. Medical innovations.   2. Medical care—Forecasting.   I. Coddington, Dean C.
   RA418.5.M4 B49 2000
   362.1—dc21   00-008789

FIRST EDITION
HB Printing   10 9 8 7 6 5 4 3 2 1

Contents

Foreword

The thesis of this book—what lies beyond managed care—may be the most important topic of our day. *We have come to the end of an old era and an old way of thinking.* The authors rightly tell us to watch for the growing role of consumers and technology—twin factors that will take center stage in the new era of health care.

There are many things to like about this book. It presents an excellent historical perspective on most of the issues that are paramount in health care today. It contains a lucid description of the contemporary health care marketplace.

Most important, it takes us beyond the present into the future. The authors suggest four scenarios that cover the waterfront of probable futures in the health care industry. Such a scope of past, present, and future is unusual in any reference work. Even better, a cord of continuity is woven through the years from 1980 to 2000 and from 2000 to 2005 that conveys a developmental perspective. We not only know where we are but how we got there and what our future is likely to be.

In addition to the extensive experience of the authors, numerous health care experts are interviewed and quoted. This provides a breadth and depth to the issues that go beyond the reach of most health care publications. Extensive use of references and an excellent bibliography complement the text.

The perspective of this book is upbeat. We have much to look forward to in the twenty-first century. Although not avoiding the tough issues we will face regarding the health care industry, the authors are optimistic about our ability to solve these problems with new and imaginative approaches. Most of us are tired of lamentation and are ready for celebration.

I love the statement in the Preface that "in this book we often refer to what are normally called health care 'costs' as 'revenue' for the health care industry." I have never been able to figure out why we celebrate when General Motors has a good year and lament when the health care industry has a good year, particularly when the local clinic or hospital may be the largest and most important employer in the community. If we truly have high value-added health care products to offer our aging population, why shouldn't we try to maximize revenues in the health care industry? After all, health care providers deal in the one product people cannot live without—life. Is that not worth more than 14 percent of the gross domestic product?

Although the book does not attempt to predict one well-defined and inevitable future for health care, it does set the stage for several alternative futures. This could be viewed as a hedge—the future is essentially unpredictable and most past efforts at forecasting have failed. However, I think the authors are demonstrating a greater wisdom than this. *They understand that the future of the health care industry depends on the choices we make today.* These should be well-informed choices and should be made from an array of alternatives. This book supplies the raw data for our choices and then invites us to make them.

We have moved from physician-managed care to third-party-managed care and are on our way to patient-managed care. Consumer empowerment via the Internet will forever change the way we deliver health care in this country. The authors' discussion of the Internet and clinical information technology alone is worth the price of this book. Any physician, clinic, hospital, or third-party agency that does not understand this revolutionary transformation is doomed.

The future is not about business as usual. It is about unusual business. It is about health care becoming an e-business. Every profession has protected its domain by restricting information to the chosen few in its profession. The Internet changes all of that. Patients have access to the same information as their physicians and will often know more about their own conditions than they did in the past. Talk about power sharing! It is about to happen in a big way.

The authors' analysis of payment system models for the future summarizes well the current thinking on the topic. The problem: I am not happy with current thinking. Why do I have to get sick to recover dollars invested in my health insurance? I don't have to die to get some value from my life insurance. I have an accumulated cash value.

The next time I go in for a flu shot, I am going to demand an MRI or maybe a bone marrow transplant. It is the only way to recover even a part of my investment. I have no financial incentive to stay well. If I am healthy, I lose all of my financial investment in my health care premiums. And while I am at it, why should I get treatment from the same folks who make the diagnosis?

What a conflict of interest! Some years ago I observed the same thing at my local auto repair shop. Stacked on the shelves were more air filters and oil filters than I had ever seen in one location. The attendant asked me if my car was running a little rough. You guessed it—he diagnosed my need for a new air filter and suggested that while he was at it we should check the oil filter as well.

Perhaps we should have freestanding health diagnostic centers that do only diagnoses and then use brokers to help us find the most cost-effective physicians and treatment facilities. Then we would be able to convert at least part of our unused health care premiums into vacations, homes, or college tuition. The authors don't bring up these possibilities, but they took the risk of asking a futurist to write the Foreword, so here they are.

I agree with the authors on the size and shape of the future health care market. We are in the middle of a boom economy, and prospects have never looked better for health care providers. It is easy to get distracted by the tribulations of the Balanced Budget Act and miss the long-term economic trend, which is clearly high growth through at least the next two decades, if not the century.

Health care providers are in the right industry at the right time. Innovative products will command premium prices. Discretionary spending in a global health care marketplace beckons. This is big-chip stuff for big players.

Although I agree with what the authors have to say in Chapter Ten about consolidation, ownership, and capacity, it is important to understand we will see a lot of disintegration as well as integration in the next few years. Most of what we have put together is not working. Our integration technology far exceeds our integration consciousness. For the most part what is required to make it all work is simply beyond us.

Virtual health care organizations own the future. They are mutable, fast, and flexible. In the human body this kind of organization is found in a neural network. We have yet to develop a comparable state of organization among physicians, hospitals, and insurance mechanisms.

All in all I highly recommend this work. It will enlighten, entertain, and challenge your current mental model of the health care industry. It is easy to read and has many convenient tables with summary data. Enjoy!

Leland Kaiser, Ph.D.
President, Kaiser Consulting

Preface

The rationalization of American healthcare is far from complete. We have only begun to inject economic discipline into healthcare.
PATRICK G. HAYS, PRESIDENT AND CEO, BLUE CROSS BLUE SHIELD ASSOCIATION, as reported by John Cochrane, *Integrated Healthcare Report*, December 1998

How do you inject economic discipline into an industry that has a split personality and conflicting financial incentives? Physicians, hospital CEOs and board members, health plan executives, and others in health care wear two hats. On the one hand, they are in the health care "business" and have the responsibility of making sure that their organizations generate revenue, are good places to work, and have a positive bottom line. The frequently quoted statement by Sister Irene Krause, board chairperson of a hospital, is apt: "No margin, no mission." On the other hand, because of the significance of health care to every American and to the country as a whole, those who earn their living in health care, or serve as voluntary board members, are stewards of a critically important public trust. They must be concerned about the high cost of health care and its impact on employers and taxpayers, about providing care for uninsured seniors and those on Medicaid, and about ensuring quality and access.

John Iglehart (1999a, p. 70), editor of *Health Affairs,* puts it this way: "In short, the American system is a work in progress, driven by a disparate array of interests with two goals that are often in conflict: providing health care to the sick and generating income for the persons and organizations that assume the financial risk."

Our Perspective in This Book

When we lament the high cost of health care—a $1.3 trillion indus-
try in the year 2000 that represents almost 14 percent of the gross
domestic product (GDP)—and its accelerating growth, we sometimes forget that this is the revenue base and livelihood for seven
hundred thousand physicians, over five million hospital employees, and over six million persons who work in other parts of health
care (including physicians' offices, health plans, manufacturing and
distribution of drugs and other health care products, association
work, consulting, and so on). The financial base of health care, in
terms of dollars loaned to hospitals and private capital invested,
represents the deployment of hundreds of billions of dollars in
financial resources.

Health care at the local level is tremendously important. The
multiple roles and impacts of health care can be seen most clearly
at the local level. As one chief financial officer (CFO) of a multihospital system in the southern part of the country told us, "What
happens in our local markets is often more important than what
goes on nationally. Don't forget; health care is a local business."

It is no exaggeration to say that physicians and local hospitals
are absolutely critical to small- and medium-sized communities in
terms of the health care services they bring. However, the jobs associated with health care, and the tie between local health care systems and opportunities for economic development, are of almost
equal importance. Furthermore, for many communities some portion of health care employment has the characteristics of a basic
industry that generates secondary jobs in other economic sectors,
such as retail, banking, and services.

At the same time local manufacturers may be competing in
national and international markets, and it is essential that their
health care costs be controlled. It is no wonder that hospital board
members—often managers and owners of local businesses—feel
like they are caught in a buzz saw.

Our focus in this book is on marketplace dynamics. We analyze
the dynamics of the health care marketplace from the perspective
of consumers and purchasers, as well as physicians and medical
groups, hospitals, integrated health care systems, and others who
deliver products and services.

In this book we often refer to what are normally called health care "costs" as "revenue" for the health care industry. We recognize health care as a huge and rapidly changing marketplace that represents tremendous opportunities for those who are leaders, or want to become leaders, in providing health care products and services. These marketplace changes also represent threats to those who do not respond.

The health care industry even now offers significant opportunities to add value. Many of the people we talk to in health care—physicians, hospital and health system CEOs, and financial officers—are uncertain about the future, both nationally and in their local markets; they are not sure their institutions will be able to adjust and survive. Furthermore, survey after survey of consumers and purchasers reveals concern, even outrage, about the current state of health care financing and delivery. With the exception of big pharmaceutical companies and some health plans, it appears that many health care organizations are dissatisfied with the current situation.

But rather than focus on the negative aspects of health care—consumers' complaints or providers' fears of funding cuts, of the growth and consolidation of managed care, and of dealing with huge losses in hospital-owned medical practices—we prefer to think of the next five years as *an era of unprecedented opportunity* for health care providers to meet customer needs. Those health care organizations that provide their customers the most value (quality, access, service, innovation, lower costs) will be the winners. We believe that opportunities to take health care to the next value-added level are breathtaking.

Why We Wrote This Book

According to a 1999 paper by Robert Mittman at the Institute for the Future, "One of the key challenges in our volatile health care environment is to plan and act based on realistic forecasts of the pace of change. Many factors conspire to make that devilishly difficult" (p. 1).

We are fully aware of the difficulties of forecasting the future of health care financing and marketplace development. However, we believe that the new millennium represents an appropriate time to identify and assess those factors most likely to influence the financing and delivery of health care in the United States.

Our objective in writing this book reminds us of Wayne Gretzky's saying that he "skates to where the puck is going, not where it is." To the extent we are successful in anticipating several possible future scenarios, we hope that the results will be beneficial to our clients, members of the Healthcare Financial Management Association (HFMA) and the Medical Group Management Association (MGMA), medical groups, hospitals, health systems, health care providers, manufacturers of health care products, employers, consumers, and policymakers.

The research and analysis that undergird *Beyond Managed Care* had two specific objectives:

- To identify and assess the factors most likely to influence the market dynamics of supply and demand for health care services in the future. These include population and income growth, the aging of the population, the growing role of consumers, the physician surplus, employers' willingness and capability to continue to provide coverage, the shape of managed care, funding for Medicare and Medicaid, the development and application of technology, and federal and state government regulations, laws, and funding levels.
- To propose four health care scenarios that attempt to address the dynamics of this marketplace. Scenario 1, incremental change, represents a continuation of what has been developing in the 1990s—expansion of managed care, increases in consumer concern about managed care, and more government regulations, such as patient protections. In scenario 4, in which retail dominates, we consider more radical changes in payment systems, such as the trend toward "defined contributions" rather than "defined benefits," the Twin Cities approach, medical savings accounts, and two different individual-insurance models.

A planned second book will pick up where this volume ends and analyze the implications and opportunities for physicians, hospitals, integrated systems, pharmaceutical companies, long-term care providers, and others who provide products and services for health care.

Research Approach

In preparing this book we relied on several sources of information. In addition to a traditional literature review, we obtained helpful information from several Web sites. We interviewed individuals with special knowledge about managed care, clinical information systems, likely breakthroughs in medical technology, consumer expectations, alternative payment systems, disease management, and government policies. Individuals interviewed are identified in the Acknowledgments.

We also relied on our experience as economic and strategy consultants to the health care industry and on the experience of one of the authors as president of the thirty-five-thousand-member Healthcare Financial Management Association (HFMA). Three of the authors are with McManis Associates. We discussed many of the issues summarized in this book with clients as three of us carried out consulting engagements, with our colleagues and with HFMA members.

The best insights into the future of managed care and of the health care system as a whole came from a series of roundtable discussions of hospital and health system CEOs, CFOs, and physicians. These panel discussions were carried out in focus group settings; we moderated and led participants in discussing many of the issues and opportunities examined in this book. A list of participants in the roundtable discussions is included in the Acknowledgments.

Denver, Colorado
June 2000

DEAN C. CODDINGTON
ELIZABETH A. FISCHER
KEITH D. MOORE
RICHARD L. CLARKE

Acknowledgments

This book involved a number of interviews, several panel discussions, a literature review, draft manuscript review, and the collaboration of a number of colleagues at McManis Associates, and the Healthcare Financial Management Association.

Roundtable Discussions and Interviews

As part of the research for this book, we conducted a number of roundtable discussions and interviews with individuals who we thought could offer insight into the future of the health care system. These included the following.

Chief Executive Officer Summit

Joel T. Allison, senior executive vice president and deputy chief executive officer, Baylor Health Care System, Dallas

J. Lindsey Bradley, chief executive officer, Trinity Mother Frances Health System, Tyler, Texas

Vince C. Caponi, chief executive officer, Central Indiana Health System, Indianapolis

Roger L. Gilbertson, M.D., president and chief executive officer, MeritCare Health System, Fargo, North Dakota

R. Timothy Stack, president and chief executive officer, Borgess Health Alliance, Kalamazoo, Michigan

Michael E. Waters, president, Hendrick Health System, Abilene, Texas

Nicholas J. Wolter, M.D., chief executive officer, Deaconess-Billings Clinic Health System, Billings, Montana

Physician Leaders

Donald C. Balfour III, M.D., chief executive officer, Sharp-Rees-Stealy Medical Group, San Diego

Laurence H. Beck, M.D., director, general internal medicine, Georgetown University Medical Center, Washington, D.C.

Joseph Gonnella, M.D., dean, Jefferson Medical College, Philadelphia

Eric Knox, M.D., chief medical officer, Obstetrix, Minneapolis

Kenneth E. Quickel Jr., M.D., president, Joslin Diabetes Center, Inc., Boston

Thomas C. Royer, M.D., president and chief executive officer, Christus Health System, Irving, Texas

Chief Financial Officers

Richard Blair, system vice president, finance and administration, Allina Health System, Minneapolis

Geraldine Hoyler, former senior vice president, finance and treasury, Catholic Health Initiatives, Denver

Thomas McNulty, senior vice president and chief financial officer, Henry Ford Health System, Detroit

Leo Lenn, corporate treasurer, Hospital Sisters Health System, Springfield, Illinois

Jay Herron, senior vice president, finance, Catholic Healthcare Partners, Cincinnati

James Combes, executive vice president and chief financial officer, Mercy Health Services, Farmington Hills, Michigan

Robert Trumpis, senior vice president, finance, Methodist Health Systems, Memphis

Peter Markell, vice president, finance, Partners HealthCare System, Inc., Boston

Public Policy

Debra S. Curtis, legislative director for Representative Forney H. "Pete" Stark (Democrat from California), Washington, D.C.

Stacey L. Hughes, senior policy adviser to Senator and Assistant Majority Leader Don Nickles (Republican from Oklahoma), Washington, D.C.

Daniel N. Mendelson, associate director for health and personnel, Office of Management and Budget, Washington, D.C.

Mary K. Wakefield, Ph.D., member of MedPAC and director of the Center for Health Policy and Ethics, George Mason University, Fairfax, Virginia

Edward J. Allera, attorney-at-law, Akin, Gump, Strauss, Hauer & Feld, LLP, Washington, D.C.

Other Individuals Interviewed

Michael Annison, president, The Westrend Group Ltd., Denver

Dennis C. Brimhall, president and associate vice chancellor, Fitzsimons–University of Colorado Health Sciences Center, Aurora, Colorado

Rufus Howe, vice president, product integration, Access Health, Broomfield, Colorado

Kris Roberts Jones, Buck Consultants

Arthur Jones, M.D., surgeon

Leland Kaiser, Ph.D., president, Kaiser & Associates, Brighton, Colorado

John Koster, M.D., vice president, clinical and physician services, Sisters of Providence Health Systems, Seattle

Steven S. Lazarus, managing principal, FHIMSS, Boundary Information Group, Denver

Greg Van Pelt, administrator of system development, Sisters of Providence, Portland, Oregon

Steve Wetzell, executive director, Buyer's Health Care Action Group, Minnetonka, Minnesota

Special Thanks

We wish to give special thanks to the following authors, executives, and consultants for their particular insights and guidance:

Sandy Lutz and E. Preston Gee, authors, *Columbia/HCA: Healthcare on Overdrive*

Regina Herzlinger, author, *Market-Driven Health Care*

The *New England Journal of Medicine,* which ran a series of articles on the U.S. health care system, including articles by John Iglehart and Robert Kuttner

The Institute for the Future, Menlo Park, California

James Hertel, founder, Healthcare Computer Corporation of America, and publisher of managed care newsletters in Colorado and Arizona

Fred Linville, VHA Mountain States

Larry Griffin, VHA Mountain States

Mark Levine, M.D., associate medical director, Colorado Foundation for Medical Care

Robert Vernon, senior vice president, Aon Managed Care

Patrick Hinton, medical group practice consultant

Anne Ladd, product manager, Micromedex, Inc.

David Buchmueller and David O'Neill, former hospital chief executive officers and executives with MMI Companies

Gerald Buckley, M.D., president, COPIC, a medical malpractice firm started by the Colorado Medical Society

Thomas Carey, M.D., cardiovascular surgeon (retired)

Allen Kortz, M.D., independent practice association member, former general surgeon

William Jobe, M.D., head of a large radiology group (retired), Denver area

Colleagues

We with to thank the following colleagues at McManis Associates and MMI:

Gerald McManis, president and chief executive officer, McManis Associates (retired)

Lou Pavia, executive vice president, McManis Associates

F. Kenneth Ackerman Jr., McManis Associates

John Misener, McManis Associates

David Stephens, McManis Associates

Lowell Palmquist, former chief executive officer, Swedish Medical Center, Englewood, Colorado, executive, VHA Inc. (retired), and part-time associate, McManis Associates

Jim Vogel, McManis Associates

Lisa Fraizer, McManis Associates

Rhonda Wyn, McManis Associates

Karen "Pete" Drury, McManis Associates

B. Frederick "Rick" Becker, chairman of St. Paul Global Healthcare

Michelle Cooney, vice president, knowledge network, St. Paul Companies

Wayne Sinclair, former senior vice president and general counsel, MMI Companies

Other Contributors

We wish to thank the following people at the Medical Group Management Association:

Cynthia Kiyotake, director, library resource center

Barry Greene, former senior vice president, education and research

Kirsten Lynam, operations manager, center for research

We wish to thank the following people at the Healthcare Financial Management Association:

Hal Prink, former director, professional development

Heather Ethridge, assistant to Dick Clarke, president

The Authors

DEAN C. CODDINGTON is a principal at McManis Associates, a health care consulting firm. After more than a decade as a research economist with the University of Denver's Research Institute, Coddington cofounded BBC Research & Consulting in 1970, which he served as a managing director for twenty-seven years before leaving to help form Moore Fischer Coddington, LLC. He received his bachelor's degree in civil engineering from South Dakota State University and his master of business administration degree from Harvard Business School. He has supervised over one hundred health care assignments for hospitals, medical groups, integrated systems, and health plans in all parts of the United States. He has coauthored five books on health care and has written numerous articles on a range of subjects, including integrated health care, factors driving health care costs, and health care strategies. Coddington is former chairman of the board of trustees of the 328-bed Swedish Medical Center in the Denver area and currently serves on the board of directors of the Colorado Neurological Institute.

ELIZABETH A. FISCHER, a principal with McManis Associates, was a founder of Moore Fischer Coddington, LLC, and before that a managing director of BBC Research & Consulting. Fischer holds a bachelor's degree in American studies and economics from Mount Holyoke College and a master's degree in city and regional planning from Harvard University. Fischer's work includes formation of hospital-affiliated group practices, product development for health plans, community needs assessment, and creation of health care networks. She also has extensive experience in rural health care and long-term care. Along with Dean C. Coddington and Keith D. Moore, she coauthored *Making Integrated Health Care Work* (Center for Research in Ambulatory Health Care Administration, 1996). She has completed more than one hundred assignments for health care organizations. She is a frequent speaker at professional meetings of various health care industry groups and coauthor of numerous articles and papers.

KEITH D. MOORE is president and chief executive officer of McManis Associates. He previously served as chairman of the board and CEO of Moore Fischer Coddington, LLC, and for fifteen years as a managing director of BBC Research & Consulting. He received his bachelor's degree in economics from the University of Texas and his master's degree in city planning from Harvard University. Moore's consulting assignments have included strategic planning, mergers of medical groups, and development of productive working relationships between physicians and hospitals. He has published several articles on health care and is coauthor, with Dean C. Coddington, of five books on health care, including *Capitalizing Medical Groups: Positioning Physicians for the Future* (McGraw-Hill, 1998). Early in his career, Moore was a senior consultant with a Denver-based consulting firm, a teaching assistant at Harvard University, and a U.S. Marine platoon leader in Vietnam. He headed the Industrial Economics and Management Division of the University of Denver's Research Institute, where he was responsible for research into technology transfer, research and development management, corporate planning, energy and resource economics, and governmental management strategies. He is a former board member of Spalding Rehabilitation Hospital in Denver.

RICHARD L. CLARKE is president of the Healthcare Financial Management Association (HFMA), headquartered in Westchester, Illinois. He is a frequent speaker at health care meetings in the United States and Europe. Clarke received his bachelor's degree in marketing and engineering from Bradley University and his master of business administration degree from the University of Miami. He earned a fellowship in HFMA in 1983. After leaving university, Clarke worked in several capacities with Jackson Memorial Hospital in Miami and then served as comptroller of Palmetto General Hospital in Hialeah, Florida. Prior to joining HFMA, Clarke was chief financial officer at Swedish Medical Center in Englewood, Colorado. He was also an active member of the Colorado chapter of HFMA and served one term as president of that organization. With Dean C. Coddington, David J. Keen, and Keith D. Moore, Clarke wrote *The Crisis in Health Care: Costs, Choices, and Strategies* (Jossey-Bass, 1990), now in its fourth printing. Along with Dean C. Coddington and Keith D. Moore, he is coauthor of *Capitalizing Medical Groups: Positioning Physicians for the Future* (McGraw-Hill, 1998).

Beyond Managed Care

Part One

Lessons Learned from the Past Two Decades

President Clinton tried to revolutionize the healthcare system in 1994, but his plan didn't get far in Congress. Nonetheless, the revolution did occur. . . . If the Clinton plan was the spark, for-profit companies were the gasoline.
SANDY LUTZ AND E. PRESTON GEE, *Columbia/HCA: Healthcare on Overdrive*, McGraw-Hill, 1998

The growth of investor-owned hospital systems, the proliferation of physician practice management companies (PPMs), and the takeover of many health plans by large insurance companies are only part of the revolution that has shaken health care in the past two decades. Other important changes have included the implementation of prospective payment for hospitals through diagnostic-related groups (DRGs), the growth of health maintenance organizations (HMOs) and preferred provider organizations (PPOs), consolidation among hospitals and health plans, and growing evidence of the importance of financial incentives in influencing physician, hospital, and health plan behavior.

The two chapters of Part One provide the historical setting for our analysis of the major factors likely to shape health care financing and the changing marketplace of the future. Chapter One deals with forces that have revolutionized the health care system as a whole, and Chapter Two focuses on the inception, growth, and influence of managed care.

Insights from the Past Two Decades

All four authors have been involved in the health care industry over the past twenty years and have personally experienced both the fundamental changes in the industry and the many fads that have initially appeared to be important but quickly turned out to be either overrated or unimportant.

Who can forget the hoopla associated with continuous quality improvement (CQI) and total quality management (TQM) or the "supermeds" of the early 1980s? (Actually, the quality movement has turned out to be important—for reasons beyond those originally anticipated—and physicians have applied these techniques in clinical process improvement.) More recently the development of provider-sponsored organizations (PSOs) was expected to create new competition for traditional HMOs and PPOs and shift more seniors into Medicare risk plans.

Many of the changes in health care over the past twenty years have been fundamental and long lasting, with their impact still being felt at the beginning of the twenty-first century. These include the long-term shift from inpatient to outpatient care, consolidation among hospitals, physicians, and health plans, explosive growth in Medicare and Medicaid, more and better (and higher-priced) drugs, the growing surplus or maldistribution of physicians, pressures on reimbursement of providers coming from managed care, the introduction and growth of new technologies, and the Balanced Budget Act (BBA) of 1997. Chapter One highlights these and other major changes of the past two decades and concludes with a summary of the implications of these changes for the future of health care.

The Changing Face of Managed Care

Most consumers and health care leaders agree that the shift away from traditional fee-for-service reimbursement and toward managed care has been the most significant trend in health care over the past two decades. In our judgment the growth of HMOs, and to a lesser extent PPOs, represents as much of a paradigm shift as the health care industry has ever experienced. Managed care is the focus of Chapter Two.

The Original HMOs

In 1980 Kaiser Permanente, Group Health Cooperative of Puget Sound in Washington, Harvard Community Health Plan (now Harvard Pilgrim Health Care), and a few other group- and staff-model HMOs were not taken very seriously. (Kaiser Permanente has been a major factor in California for more than fifty years, but prior to 1980 HMOs represented small players in big ponds.) HMOs were viewed as "an interesting experiment" coming out of the Nixon administration's efforts to control health care costs. HMO doctors were in the minority and not considered to be in the mainstream of medicine.

The broader HMO movement has seen enrollment increase sevenfold since 1980, and these types of health plans now serve just under half of the employees of companies that offer health insurance coverage as well as those employees' families. When HMO participants in Medicare and Medicaid are added, more than one-quarter of the country's population was served by HMOs in 2000.

The Advent of PPOs

PPOs have had their ups and downs over the past two decades but continue to be major players in the health care industry. Although the first PPOs date back to the late 1970s, these types of health plans did not emerge as serious players until the mid-1980s. From 1985 to 1990 PPOs were often dismissed as a transitional payment system useful primarily in preparing consumers for the more rigorous limitations imposed by tightly managed HMOs.

To the surprise of many, PPOs are still around and going strong. As the 1990s drew to a close, consumers became more resistant to the gatekeeper requirements of many HMOs and showed their dislike for the limited panels of physicians offered by these types of health plans by opting for point-of-service (POS) plans and PPOs. The complexities of moving more aggressively into the capitated payment of physicians and hospitals—paying them a fixed amount per member per month—have also slowed the growth of HMOs. PPOs, however, do not use primary care gatekeepers, do not normally pay physicians on a capitated basis, usually offer larger panels of physicians, and are not as complicated to organize and manage. As of the year 2000 it was estimated that PPOs were available to more than 40 percent of all workers of organizations offering health care benefits. This equates to one-quarter of all Americans.

The Future of Managed Care

Managed care has grown from the equivalent of a corporate start-up to a mature industry in less than fifteen years. An important question, and one that relates to the title of this book, is, What lies beyond managed care as we know it today? The answer: major change, especially in scenario 4.

To chart the future course of managed care, we begin by looking back over the past two decades at the forces shaping the U.S. health care marketplace and their implications for the future.

Chapter One

Twenty Years of Health Care Revolution

A Look Back

It's hard not to be impressed by the sweep of change, both in the capabilities of the American health system and in health care organizations, over the last 20 years.

JEFF GOLDSMITH, "Operation Restore Human Values," *Hospitals and Health Networks,* July 1998

Jeff Goldsmith, a well-known speaker and author, has recognized the speed and magnitude of change in the health care industry. He remarks, "In the space of a single generation, health services have evolved from a cottage industry into a substantial corporate enterprise. A breathtaking array of new technologies have been added to the hospital's diagnostic and therapeutic capability. Hospitals have also managed—though not always gracefully—the transition to a more ambulatory and community-based model of care" (Goldsmith, 1998a, p. 74).

This chapter takes a detailed look at what has happened in the health care marketplace over the past twenty years. The time line shown in Figure 1.1 identifies a number of shocks to the health care system that occurred during the period from 1980 through 1999.

Probably the biggest jolt to the old way of doing things came when the Health Care Financing Administration (HCFA) introduced prospective payment through diagnostic-related groups in 1983. This effort to take hospitals out of purely fee-for-service reimbursement and force accountability on both hospitals and physicians (hospitals could not survive DRGs without the cooperation

---

Figure 1.1. Major Developments in the
U.S. Health Care System, 1980–1999.

1980　State rate review boards attempt to control hospital costs

Era of expansion among hospitals continues

HMO enrollment reaches ten million

1981　Traditional indemnity insurance and fee-for-service medicine dominate

Diversification strategies are popular

1982　Medical services inflation exceeds 10 percent

1983　VHA becomes more aggressive in expanding membership in alliance

HCFA institutes prospective payment (DRGs)

Proprietary hospital system boom (HCA, NME, AMI, and Humana)

1984　HCA acquires Welsey Medical Center in Wichita, Kansas

Inpatient days begin long-term decline

Era of competition in health care begins

1985　Aetna and VHA form Partners National Health Plans

For-profits get into health plan business (Humana Plus)

PPOs begin to develop

First laparoscopic surgery

1986　MRIs become common

HMOs exceed twenty million lives covered

1987　Certificate of need legislation ends in most states

Rick Scott establishes Columbia

PhyCor established

1988　PhyCor leads to a boom in PPMs

Medicare spending reaches $100 billion

1989　Double-digit annual increases in health care costs

RBRVS established

---

of physicians) played a big part in the introduction of competition, price cutting, and Wall Street capital into the health care industry. The combination of DRGs, increased competition, and the growth of managed care equaled a mid-1980s paradigm shift that is still being played out. Exhibit 1.1 summarizes the major factors that have shaped health care over the past two decades and that have implications for the future.

The Role of Financial Incentives

When we look back, we are struck by the importance of financial incentives, and changes to these incentives, in shaping the health care marketplace of the past two decades.

1990	Medical group consolidation begins in earnest
1991	CQI comes on strong in hospitals
1992	Vertical integration strategy popular
	Medicare enrollment reaches thirty-five million
1993	Clinton health care reform task force publishes report
	PHOs pick up steam
1994	Clinical information system development begins in earnest
	Columbia has 311 hospitals in thirty-one states
1995	Gene research and DNA testing are highly publicized
	Interest in clinical guidelines gains momentum
	Marshfield antitrust case begins
	HMO enrollment passes fifty million
1996	HMOs come under attack for restricting care
	Columbia is the tenth largest employer in the United States
	Managed care passes one hundred million lives covered
1997	Corporate compliance becomes a major initiative
	Kaiser Permanente loses $270 million
	BBA becomes law
	Columbia/HCA executives are indicted; Scott resigns
	Prudential and Aetna sell physician practices
1998	Bust in PPM boom; MedPartners divests itself of medical groups
	Y2K efforts intensify
	AHERF system in Pittsburgh and Philadelphia goes bankrupt
	Health care passes $1 trillion in revenues
1999	Number of uninsured reaches forty-four million
	Some BBA relief

DRGs, the Resource-Based Relative Value Scale, and Medicare HMOs

Changes in financial incentives include the advent of DRGs for hospital inpatient services, changes in the way physicians are paid by HCFA through the Resource-Based Relative Value Scale (RBRVS), capitation of primary care physicians (paying a fixed amount per member per month), global capitation (including most medical services), and the shifting of Medicare recipients to HMOs.

Each of these departures from traditional fee-for-service medicine has had important ramifications. DRGs forced physicians and hospitals to look more closely at how they were using resources—staffing, facilities, and supplies—in managing patients. Capitated

Exhibit 1.1. Highlights of the Past Two Decades: Implications for the Future.

- The consolidation of hospitals, medical groups, and health plans has been one of the most visible signs of change in health care over the past twenty years, and it is likely to continue.
- The injection of Wall Street capital into hospitals, medical groups, and health plans often had a destabilizing effect.
- The shifting of risk to physicians and hospitals during the past two decades will change; risk will be passed on to consumers.
- The technological change, including new drugs, characterizing the past twenty years is a preview of what is to come in the first five years of the new millennium.
- The decline in inpatient care and the growth of outpatient services that emerged in the early 1980s will accelerate in the future.
- Growth in the number of the uninsured and those on Medicaid represents an untenable factor threatening the future of many hospitals and medical groups.
- The success of vertical integration, popular in the mid-1990s, has been spotty at best. However, there is a continuing need for coordinated care and for physicians and hospitals to work together.
- The financial incentives of the health care marketplace—a mix of capitated and fee-for-service payment—continue to be inconsistent, and the hybrid payment system is dysfunctional.

payment of primary care physicians influenced referral patterns to specialists and turned financial incentives in the opposite direction (less is better under capitation).

Here are examples of how the payment system has affected the use of hospitals:

- When DRGs were phased in during the period from 1983 to 1985, there was an immediate and continuing drop in average length of stay in most hospitals in the United States.
- In California and other states with widespread managed care providing capitated payment for primary care physicians and some specialists, the average number of inpatient days per thousand residents (commercial) dropped by two-thirds.

- For Medicare patients in an HMO setting, the average number of inpatient days per thousand enrollees dropped by more than half from the late 1980s to the early 1990s.

Shift to Outpatient Services

Much of the shift from inpatient to outpatient surgery has been driven by technology, changes in reimbursement, and consumer preferences. In the early 1980s insurance companies were not generous payers for outpatient diagnostic and surgical procedures; it was financially beneficial for both physicians and hospitals to have these procedures performed on an inpatient basis. However, this scenario began to change in the mid-1980s, and the evidence of a massive shift from inpatient to outpatient procedures is overwhelming (see Figure 1.2).

Figure 1.2. Trends in Community Hospital Inpatient Days and Outpatient Visits.

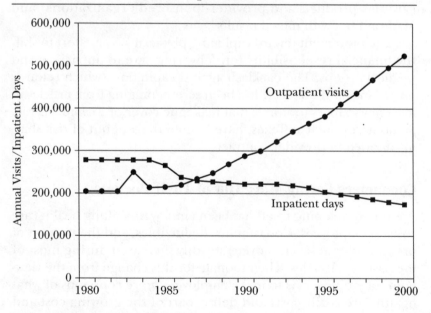

Sources: American Hospital Association (1993, p. 7, tab. 1; 1996, p. 3, tab. 1); authors' estimates for 1997–2000.

Mixed Financial Incentives

Health care ended the twentieth century with a complex, confusing, and often dysfunctional payment system—mostly discounted fee-for-service for physicians (but with some capitation) and DRGs, per diems, and fee-for-service for hospitals. This payment system sends mixed messages to health care providers. As one physician leader told us, "Managing today is like driving a car with one foot on the accelerator (fee-for-service) and one on the brake (capitation). Also, we don't know whether to look out the rear window to see who is coming after us or look through the windshield to identify the hazards in the road ahead."

Shifting Risk to Physicians and Hospitals

One theme of the past two decades has been the shift of insurance risk to physicians and hospitals and away from managed care and health insurance companies. As the 1990s drew to a close, HCFA was trying the same approach with Medicare (for example, Medicare risk products and provider-sponsored organizations) and Medicaid but with mixed results.

The movement toward capitating physicians is an effort to shift the financial responsibility for delivering care to physicians and medical groups. The backlash against capitation (which rewards physicians for doing less) has been severe, ranging from articles in local newspapers to stories that make the cover of *Time* magazine. Some states, such as Texas, have limited the amount of risk sharing allowed in provider contracts.

Consumers Paying More Out of Their Pockets

Another developing trend has been employers shifting health care costs to employees. Copayments, deductibles, and the portion of premiums paid by employees steadily increased during most of the past two decades. The rationale for this change from the viewpoint of employers is to make employees more conscious of what health care really costs and defray part of the growing cost and expansion of health care benefits. This shift is a harbinger of things to come, especially the trend toward "defined contributions" rather than "defined benefits" (discussed in detail in Chapter Twelve).

Tapping Discretionary Income and Gains in Wealth

There is another aspect of consumers increasing their share of total health care spending. A growing number of consumers are paying for the medical procedures and products they want, and they are paying big—far more than anyone would have anticipated just a few years ago.

Examples of discretionary consumer spending include cosmetic surgery, which has experienced phenomenal growth in the past three years. Certain types of long-term care—congregate care and assisted living—have grown rapidly despite the lack of insurance coverage or government payment sources. The same type of growth is evident in the amount spent on complementary and alternative treatments, such as acupuncture, herbs, chiropractic, and other nontraditional approaches.

The Boom in Pharmaceuticals

Drug companies have capitalized on a strong economy and consumers' willingness to pay for health care products by offering a wide array of lifestyle drugs (for example, Viagra and Rogaine). Health plans and Medicare do not normally cover the cost of these drugs, but consumers are buying them anyway.

Their advertising on television and in national magazines like *Newsweek* and *Sports Illustrated* demonstrates pharmaceutical manufacturers' desire to market directly to consumers. This marketing strategy is working, and the pharmaceutical costs of most health plans are out of control. A physician who is the medical director of a large HMO told us, "There is no way that health plans should be getting into the business of offering more financial assistance for consumers to purchase drugs. As much as some of these drugs are needed, and help people, we would go broke in a New York minute if we began to expand pharmaceutical benefits."

Shifting the Risks of Health Care Costs to Consumers

Whereas one of the trends clearly established in the 1980s and 1990s was the shift in the risk of paying for health care from insurance companies and government programs to physicians and hospitals, the next big shift will be to consumers. This is coming in the form of defined contributions rather than defined benefits for consumers. We have much more to say about this developing trend throughout most of the remainder of this book.

Health Care Industry Consolidation

There has been significant consolidation in almost every segment of health care: health plans, hospitals, physicians and medical groups, specialty hospitals, rehabilitation, drug companies, and long-term care.

Health Plan Consolidation

It is evident that health plans have consolidated at a rapid pace over the past five years. However, if we look back to 1980, the health plan industry was even more consolidated; the various statewide Blue Cross and Blue Shield (BCBS) systems covered the vast majority of the population.

Beginning in the early 1980s, we witnessed extraordinary fragmentation of health plan coverage patterns. But by the mid-1990s the health plan industry was consolidating at a rapid pace, led by BCBS systems, such as Anthem in Indiana and Trigon in Virginia, and by several of the large insurance companies, such as Aetna U.S. Healthcare and CIGNA. With declining profits in the late 1990s, health plans sought greater scale in order to spread fixed costs and wield greater market influence.

Hospital Consolidation

Looking back over the past twenty years, there have been two waves of hospital consolidation. The first was in the early to mid-1980s, when four "proprietary" systems—American Medical International

(AMI), Hospital Corporation of American (HCA), National Medical Enterprises (NME), and Humana—grew rapidly, mainly through acquisitions. By the mid-1990s, however, these four systems had virtually disappeared, to be replaced by Columbia/HCA and Tenet. For example, Humana sold its hospitals to Galen, which sold to Columbia before Columbia acquired HCA.

Hospital consolidation is not limited to investor-owned companies. We estimate that three-fourths of the mergers and acquisitions of the past five years have involved not-for-profit multihospital systems and community hospitals.

The two large hospital alliances, VHA Inc. and Premier, have been adding members during the past two decades. VHA has grown from fewer than one hundred hospitals in 1980 to over fifteen hundred by the end of 1999. Premier has over one thousand hospitals in the alliance, many in multihospital systems. These alliances provide a variety of services, including group purchasing.

As the curtain fell on the decade of the 1990s, it appeared that Columbia/HCA and several other investor-owned hospital management companies (such as Tenet and Quorum) lacked the potential for significant future growth. Stock prices were down, and the ability to improve profits through consolidation were unproven. However, we can expect more acquisition and merger activity among not-for-profit systems like Catholic Health Initiatives, Sutter in California, and Baptist Health System in Alabama.

Physician and Medical Group Consolidation

The consolidation of physicians and medical groups has been proceeding at a rapid rate over the past two decades. The proportion of physicians in solo practice dropped from close to half in 1980 to less than a quarter in 2000. The percentage of doctors who are employees has grown from around 20 percent in 1980 to 45 percent at the end of the 1990s (estimates based on American Medical Association data; see Cochrane, 1999a, p. 4). At the same time the consolidation of physicians in independent practice associations (IPAs), physician-hospital organizations (PHOs), and other types of "virtual" organizations, or networks, has been one of the outstanding stories of the past two decades.

Other Aspects of Health Care Consolidation

The physician practice management industry was one approach to consolidating physician practices. At their peak in 1998 there were over thirty publicly owned PPMs and another three hundred in their formative stages. As some of the large PPMs unraveled in the late 1990s, many of the physicians in medical groups that were acquired and then spun off continued to stay together. HealthSouth is an example of a publicly owned firm that has consolidated rehabilitation and outpatient surgery services. Many drug companies have merged or been acquired. There have been large systems built in mental health; however, several of these have run into hard times. There appears to be little doubt that health care industry consolidation will continue to be strong during the first five years of the twenty-first century (this is discussed in greater detail in Chapter Ten).

Physician-Hospital Integration

Interest on the part of physicians and hospitals in working together in new and creative ways has been one of the benefits of the growth of managed care. In the early 1990s this was reflected in the formation of hundreds of PHOs, which exist primarily for the purpose of "single-signature contracting" (one entity authorized to enter into managed care contracts for both a physician organization and hospital). During this period many hospital CEOs and physician leaders were excited about "going after the premium dollar."

What Is Physician-Hospital Integration?

This question is not as easy to answer as it might seem. Figure 1.3 depicts our definition of vertical integration of physicians, hospitals, and health plans. Not all vertically integrated systems contain every element shown in the figure. However, the major distinguishing factor of an integrated system is an organized effort on the part of physicians and a hospital or multihospital system to work in partnership to coordinate patient care.

Has Vertical Integration Reached Its Peak?

Interest in vertical integration reached a high point in the mid-1990s and was coming under increasing criticism as the 1990s

Figure 1.3. Components of Integrated Health Care Systems.

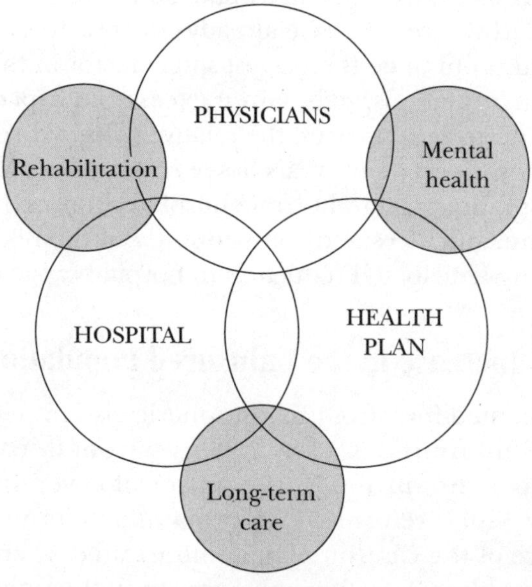

came to an end. However, we believe that the lessons learned from the more sophisticated vertically integrated systems—most led by multispecialty clinics—continue to be valuable in understanding the potential for cooperation and coordination in health care. The more advanced integrated systems, such as Marshfield in Wisconsin, Geisinger in Pennsylvania, and Intermountain Health Care in Utah, have been leaders in developing primary care networks, clinical information systems, clinical guidelines, and "seamless," or coordinated, systems of care.

Balanced Budget Act of 1997

An increasing number of hospital CEOs, physician leaders, and experts on the health care industry are saying that the new rules and financial limitations imposed by the federal government's Balanced Budget Act represented the most significant new external factor influencing health care in the late 1990s and that the significance of the BBA may extend into the twenty-first century. (These comments echo those we heard in 1983 when DRGs were introduced.)

There is little doubt that restrictions on reimbursement represent a serious threat to the future financial viability of many hospitals, particularly those that have already cut costs to the bone. The BBA could turn out to be the biggest single factor in the closure of financially marginal hospitals. Given excess bed capacity and the shift toward outpatient services, the relatively slow rate of closure of hospitals over the past twenty years has been a surprise. Many experts were wrong in forecasting wholesale hospital closures due to DRGs, managed care, and increased competition. But the BBA may bring about the long-anticipated reduction in hospital capacity.

Continued Increase in the Uninsured Population

With an estimated forty-five million Americans (16 percent of the population) uninsured in early 2000 (up from thirty-seven million, or 14 percent, in 1993), the universal coverage discussed during the Clinton reform efforts remains an elusive target. But as the failure of the Clinton plan demonstrated, there is no easy fix for this problem. Of course, the growth in the uninsured population places increased pressures on physicians and hospitals to provide "charity care." However, largely because of the financial impact of the BBA, many smaller hospitals and those in urban areas with a heavy Medicare base have lost much of their ability to care for the uninsured. From the viewpoint of physicians and hospitals this is a problem that has been growing steadily worse over the past two decades and is now reaching crisis proportions. There is growing evidence that the uninsured, most of whom hold jobs, are not receiving good-quality health care (see Chapter Eleven). The large and growing number of the uninsured is one indication of the "dysfunctional" nature of the health care industry.

Medical Technology and Information Systems

Nearly every health care industry observer, the authors of this book included, cites technology as one of the two or three most important factors influencing health care costs and quality over the past two decades.

Examples of New Medical Technologies

What are some examples of technology that has affected health care? Advances in open-heart surgery and all that goes with it—heart-lung pumps, cardiac catheterization labs, and angioplasty procedures—are one example. In the early 1980s these procedures were limited to tertiary care hospitals; today open-heart surgery is performed at many smaller hospitals.

Laparoscopic surgery, developed in Germany in 1985, had important implications, especially for gallbladder surgery. One surgeon who was trained in this procedure in the early 1990s said, "We didn't have any choice; the consumers demanded it. If you proposed to take out a gallbladder the old-fashioned way, they went to another surgeon." Laparoscopic surgery has been widely used in the United States for gallbladder removal since 1988. By 1993 more than half a million laparoscopic gallbladder surgeries had been performed. Other surgical applications for laparoscopic technology include thoracic, pediatric, gynecological, urological, orthopedic, plastic, and ear, nose, and throat surgery (Eubanks and Schauer, 1996, p. 791).

Another physician, who has been in private practice for over thirty years, said that, without a doubt, from a diagnostic viewpoint computerized tomography (CT) scanning, magnetic resonance imaging (MRI), and ultrasound have been extremely important developments. "These new technologies cut down on the need for exploratory surgeries and enable physicians to do a better diagnostic job." The same physician said that he puts laser surgery, especially for the eyes, in the category of one of the most important technological breakthroughs of the past two decades.

New Drugs and Other Therapies

One doctor of internal medicine, who has been in practice for thirty-five years, told us that the most important development in medicine in his years of practice has been effective drugs for treating hypertension. His comment bears out what the medical literature has been saying: it is the application of drugs and technology that has had the biggest impact on the lives of patients.

Investment in Information Technology

The development of clinical and management information systems, which began in earnest in the early 1990s, has consumed billions of dollars of health care earnings and reserves, with few benefits to either consumers or health care organizations. Continuing investment on an even more massive scale seems certain. It would be a mistake, however, to consider these large investments in information technology to be an error or of marginal potential benefit. We believe the future payoff of these huge investments is one of the most exciting changes that will influence how health care is financed and delivered in the twenty-first century and beyond. (Clinical information systems are discussed in more detail in Chapter Eight.)

Continuous Quality Improvement and Clinical Guidelines

Continuous quality improvement and clinical guidelines have a related and interesting history of ups and downs in the health care industry. Sometimes derided as "cookbook medicine," clinical guidelines had become widely accepted by the end of the twentieth century. CQI was all the rage in hospitals in the late 1980s and early 1990s. The pioneering work of W. Edwards Deming became the mantra of most of the leading hospitals in the country. The Joint Committee on the Accreditation of Healthcare Organizations (JCAHO) built CQI principles into its accreditation criteria. CQI consulting firms and gurus, like the Juran Group, Crosby, and Dr. Donald Berwick, were in high demand and commanded premium rates. Hospital administrators and others became "coaches," and most employees were on the "team." Quality circles were common. The remnants of the CQImovement are still present in many organizations.

But with hospitals taking the lead in CQI, there were initial concerns about how physicians might react. In the early days there was often little physician involvement in CQI, and most of the processes analyzed and improved were administrative in nature, such as admissions processing, staff scheduling, and food service.

However, during the late 1980s and early 1990s, physicians began to take note of the potential for CQI in reducing variation among clinical processes. Brent James of Intermountain Health Care (IHC), an international expert on improving quality, is an example. Most physicians recognize that clinical variation is rampant among medical specialists on the same medical staff or in the same group and between communities. This has been made evident over the past twenty years by the valuable research of John Wennberg of Dartmouth and his studies of clinical variation among comparable towns in New England and other locales.

The implications of CQI and its adaptation to clinical guideline development are profound for the future of health care, especially managed care. With an increasing number of physicians and medical groups using guidelines, the need for second-guessing and concurrent review and control of referrals to specialists and hospitals diminishes dramatically. Thus one of the most objectionable features of managed care from the viewpoint of physicians—the second-guessing of clinical and patient care decisions by outside reviewers, who are usually not physicians—may be eliminated.

Other Themes of the Past Two Decades

There are a number of other important changes that came about in the 1990s, including the growth of the Medicare population, increased oversight of physicians and hospitals, and the changing role of primary care physicians.

Growing Number of People on Medicare

This has not been a sudden shock to the health care system but instead a continuous trend that is about to reach dramatic proportions. More than half a million Americans reach Medicare age each year, and the aging of the population is leading to tremendous increases in demand for health care services. And the best (if you are a provider), or the worst (if you are the federal government or a taxpayer), is yet to come. The growth in the Medicare population over the past twenty years, including the disabled, is shown in Figure 1.4.

Figure 1.4. Medicare Enrollment Trends, 1980–2000.

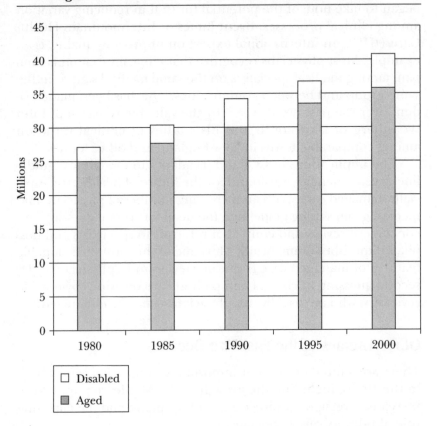

Sources: Health Care Financing Administration, 1999; authors' estimates for 2000.

Increased Payer Oversight

Physicians and hospitals have noticed this payer oversight from two major sources: managed care plans and HCFA. There is hardly a medical group, hospital, or other type of health care organization that has not implemented a corporate compliance program aimed at staying out of trouble with HCFA and other payers. The Columbia/HCA debacle that hit in mid-1997 led to an acceleration of this trend, and it will undoubtedly spill over into the next five years. Of course, payer oversight on the clinical side is the biggest single source of annoyance and dissatisfaction among physicians. The looking over shoulders and second-guessing by managed care plans that reached its zenith in the 1990s has alienated a large proportion of practicing physicians from managed care.

Changing Role of Primary Care

In the early 1980s, during the heyday of fee-for-service medicine and freedom to choose any physician or hospital, primary care physicians were not a strong force in health care. (There were some exceptions, including Kaiser Permanente and several large multispecialty clinics.) But with the growth of HMOs in the mid-1980s, along with their emphasis on primary care gatekeepers, primary care physicians became the darlings of health care.

By 1993, at the time of the Clinton health care reform proposal, there was widespread agreement that the country had too few primary care physicians (general internists, pediatricians, family practice physicians, and obstetrician gynecologists) and a growing surplus of medical specialists. Many medical schools began to adjust their ratios of primary care physicians (PCPs) to specialists.

However, as the 1990s came to a close and consumers were making known their preference for PPO and POS plans, HMOs were backing off on the gatekeeper concept, thus reducing the influence of PCPs. At the same time the supply of PCPs appears to have caught up with demand in many communities.

Local Focus

While focusing on national trends and change factors, we must not forget that health care is a local industry. A small town with a twenty-bed hospital that loses its only physician to retirement or death and cannot replace this beloved doctor has experienced just as severe a shock to its local health care system as a metropolitan area that undergoes a change to managed care.

In a two-hospital town, the local health care system will panic when two medical groups merge, join a PPM firm, and decide to take most of their business to one hospital rather than split it down the middle. The departure or retirement of a longtime hospital administrator can be a shock to a small hospital and the community.

The shutdown of a 150-employee manufacturing plant and the subsequent loss of jobs that provided health benefits is serious from both an economic and a health care viewpoint.

In some small communities county governments subsidize the local hospital and nursing home (they are often co-owned and comanaged). If an oil-producing county runs into financial difficulties, say, because of a drop in oil prices, this can represent a serious threat to the economic viability of the local hospital.

The revolution in health care and the shocks to the system often look quite different from a local perspective. The need to cope with local problems and issues often occupies most of the time and energy of community hospital boards, hospital managers, and physician leaders.

Patterns of Change with Important Implications for the Future

We believe there are several patterns emerging from this review of the past two decades, and many of these are likely to influence the shape of the health care marketplace over the first five years of the new millennium. Here are our nominees for the most important:

1. *Consolidation.* The consolidation of hospitals, physicians, medical groups, health plans, home health providers, long-term care facilities, and other medical services (such as dentistry, rehabilitation, and vision care) has been one of the most visible signs of change in health care over the past two decades. The results are mixed, with more questionable outcomes than clear-cut successes.

Consolidation will most likely continue over the next few years. Whether it results in significant benefits for patients and payers remains to be seen.

2. *Capital investment.* It is difficult to reconcile the demands of Wall Street with those of the three key sectors of health care: the medical group, the hospital, and the health plan.

The experience of the past two decades suggests that the injection of Wall Street capital into the key elements of health care has not generally paid off for long-term investors and has had a destabilizing effect on many communities.

3. *Shifting of financial risk to consumers.* The trend of the 1980s and 1990s has been to shift the risk of financing health care to providers—physicians, medical groups, and hospitals. This trend will continue but will not be the most important one with respect to the shifting of financial risk in the future. (This issue is especially important in scenario 4, described in Chapter Thirteen.)

> *The dominant trend of the next decade will be to shift*
> *an increasing amount of financial risk to consumers.*

4. *Technology and research.* The proliferation of technology and new drugs has affected the way health care is delivered, but this represents the tip of the iceberg compared with what we can expect over the next few years. Research into the genetic makeup of humans promises revolutionary changes. Internet access to medical information for both consumers and providers will have profound ramifications. (These points constitute scenario 3, described in Chapter Thirteen.)

> *We expect unprecedented change from the impact of genetic research,*
> *new drugs, and medical technology over the next five years.*

5. *Information technology.* Health care information technology (IT), clinical guidelines, and outcomes measures are finally beginning to realize their potential. The 1990s was an era of heavy investment in these approaches, and we expect this to continue into the new century.

> *The next five years may be a time for a limited number of health*
> *care organizations to begin to harvest the benefits of past financial*
> *commitments to IT.*

6. *Increase in outpatient care.* Although consumers are generally pleased with the shift from inpatient to outpatient care, it poses continuing challenges to the economic viability of many hospitals. This trend will continue to be a factor for both consumers and providers.

> *The long-term trend away from inpatient admissions toward*
> *outpatient services will continue.*

7. *Growing ranks of the uninsured.* The forty-five million uninsured Americans, added to the thirty million on Medicaid, amount to one-fourth of the U.S. population. The substantial size of the uninsured population has significant implications for the future of health care. (See Chapter Five for more discussion of this issue.)

The growing ranks of the uninsured represent a destabilizing factor for the future of health care financing and delivery.

8. *Integration and coordinated care.* Although the history of vertical integration and coordinated care is spotty at best and many hospital boards and CEOs are losing confidence in the strategy, we expect more success stories to emerge in the next few years to offset widely publicized failures, thus giving vertical integration a needed boost.

Vertical integration, along with disease management, continues to hold promise for the seamless (coordinated) delivery of health care services.

9. *Contradictory financial incentives.* Prior to DRGs and the growth spurt of HMOs, financial incentives were generally aligned around fee-for-service medicine. Of course, this caused health care costs to skyrocket. But the present mixed system of discounted fee-for-service, per diem rates for hospitals, and capitation for physicians is untenable. At one time it was believed that capitation was synonymous with HMOs and that the growth of HMOs would make capitation the dominant payment mechanism. This has not happened, and we have a hybrid payment system that is dysfunctional. (Imagine being a physician with one-quarter of your patients uninsured or on Medicaid, one-quarter enrolled in an HMO that pays on a capitated basis, one-quarter in a PPO that pays on a discounted fee-for-service basis, and one-quarter on Medicare!)

The financial incentives of the health care marketplace continue to be inconsistent and dysfunctional.

Having made these observations about many of the major shocks that have revolutionized the health care marketplace over the past two decades and having outlined the implications of these change factors for the future, we move on to the main story of the past two decades: the growth of managed care.

Chapter Two

The Maturing of Managed Care

Managed care sneaked up on physicians; by the time they fully grasped the implications, it was a fait accompli.
ROBERT KUTTNER, "Must Good HMOs Go Bad? The Commercialization of Prepaid Group Health Care," *New England Journal of Medicine*, 1998

In the 1980s managed care caught many physicians by surprise. However, by the mid-1990s most physicians, even those practicing in some of the more remote regions of the United States, had first-hand experience with managed care. Over 90 percent of all physicians are part of a group practice, IPA, or PHO that has at least one managed care contract.

Although physicians' attitudes toward managed care are critically important, and are discussed later, this chapter is much broader in scope. Here we summarize the origins of HMOs and PPOs, their initial objectives, their growth (and the corresponding decline of traditional indemnity insurance), the impact of managed care on quality and costs, "community" versus "experience" rating, "cherry picking," and issues of consumer choice and satisfaction. We conclude this chapter with several observations about the future of managed care, especially as it relates to our four scenarios for the future.

Figure 2.1 shows the growth in managed care in the United States from 1980 to 2000. The graph presents the number of employees and their family members enrolled in commercial HMOs,

Medicaid, and Medicare HMOs and eligible for PPOs. In 2000 the total number of HMO subscribers exceeded seventy-two million, including those in Medicare and Medicaid risk plans. Employees and their families eligible for PPO services accounted for another seventy-three million. By 2000 managed care had been chosen by just over half of all Americans and was available to two-thirds of the population.

Exhibit 2.1 highlights the major findings of this chapter, with an emphasis on implications for the future of managed care.

**Figure 2.1. Growth in Managed Care
in the United States, 1980–2000.**

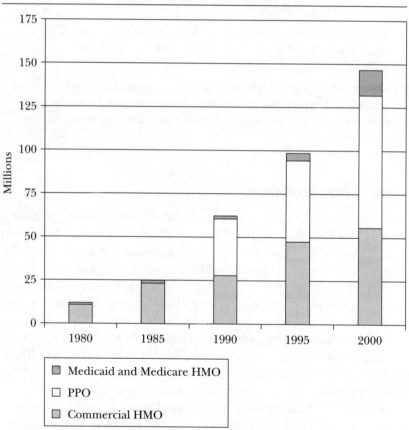

Note: As of January 1 of each year.
Sources: InterStudy, 1997, pp. v–viii; authors' estimates.

**Exhibit 2.1. The Maturing of Managed Care:
Implications for the Future.**

- Capitation as a payment mechanism for physicians and medical groups has topped out.

- Managed care serves 85 percent of the employees who work for employers offering health benefits; it is a mature industry.

- Without new life in Medicare risk products, the growth potential of HMOs is limited.

- HMOs have loosened their restrictions, most notably the need to go through a primary care gatekeeper. Even with this shift, recent managed care growth has been in PPOs and open-access plans, not in traditional HMOs.

- The number of individuals covered by employer-based health insurance declined from 156 million in 1990 to 141 million in 2000.

- The founding principles of managed care—prevention, early detection of disease, coordination of care, and cost-effectiveness—appear to be as relevant today as when they were first articulated by Henry Kaiser and Paul Ellwood.

What Is Managed Care?

Here is the definition of managed care used in one industry report (HCIA, 1998, p. ix): "Managed care is a broad term that encompasses the type of care provided by various kinds of health maintenance organizations (HMOs), preferred provider organizations (PPOs), and other health plans that assume insurance risk and practice selective contracting (limiting enrollees to a panel of providers) and some type of utilization review. Managed care combines the delivery and finance aspects of health care." There are significant regional variations in how managed care is defined. In California, for example, managed care usually refers to HMOs and capitated (PMPM) payment of physicians. However, in most other regions, managed care is defined more broadly to include PPOs. Our definition of managed care? Nothing complicated: HMOs and PPOs.

The First HMO: The Kaiser Story

The history of HMOs began with Henry Kaiser, a West Coast ship-builder and industrialist. (For the source of the Kaiser story as presented here, see Kaiser Industries, 1984.)

Henry Kaiser's Early Experience with Health Care

In a 1965 speech Henry Kaiser told how his mother died in his arms when he was sixteen. "We were poor. We could not afford a doctor nor the hospital care which could have saved her life. I resolved then and there to do something about people dying for lack of medical care" (Kaiser Industries, 1984, p. 55).

Sidney Garfield Enters the Scene

In 1933 more than five thousand men were cutting a canal to carry fresh water from the Colorado River to Los Angeles. If any of these workers were hurt or sick, they faced a two-hundred-mile trip to Los Angeles. This presented an opportunity to a young surgeon named Sidney Garfield. He organized a small team of physicians and with $2,500 built a twelve-bed hospital.

By 1938 the construction camps along the aqueduct had closed and Garfield was back in private practice in Los Angeles, when a Kaiser-sponsored team was the successful bidder in the Grand Coulee project in Washington. Although there was a hospital near the Grand Coulee site, the labor unions were dissatisfied, and Edgar Kaiser asked for the opportunity to run the hospital. Garfield was available and accepted the task.

As the number of workers and family members reached five thousand, Henry Kaiser convinced the partners in the Grand Coulee project to prepay the cost of industrial accidents; workers prepaid $0.07 a day for other medical care. Later their wives were included for an additional $0.07 a day and children for $0.25 a week. Commenting on the success of this pioneering health care system, one of the doctors said, "People came to the hospital with early symptoms. There wasn't the factor of medical cost to keep them away. They could come with the first pain in their abdomen, when they first felt their colds, when we could catch the appendix before it ruptured, and would get their pneumonia cases before they were terminal. We would take care of them and they would get well" (Kaiser Industries, 1984, p. 57). (This resembles present-day arguments in favor of universal coverage!)

Prepaid Plan Comes to the Bay Area

After the Pearl Harbor attack, employment at the Kaiser shipyards in the Bay Area jumped to thirty thousand, inundating the area's already overtaxed medical facilities. The doctors from Grand Coulee were called in to organize a medical plan. Henry Kaiser created a nonprofit foundation called Permanente, separate from the Kaiser industrial organization, to finance the new plan. The medical program began in April 1942 and eventually covered a wartime workforce of two hundred thousand. However, when World War II ended, the number of workers dropped to thirty-two thousand. A question then arose: Should the prepaid medical program continue?

Postwar Decision to Move Forward

The former members of the wartime plan represented a powerful force for keeping the plan alive. The physicians themselves had found the advantages of prepaid group practice to their liking and wanted to continue. The major issue was one of economics: Would such a program be able to compete against other established medical insurance plans and be economically viable?

Henry Kaiser tipped the scales, remembering his vow from the time of his mother's death. He told his wavering associates, "Well, here's our chance, boys" (Kaiser Industries, 1984, p. 59). The challenge was accepted, and enrollment was opened to groups and individuals on a voluntary basis. To ensure that no one could be forced to join this type of plan, all prospective membership groups were required to offer an alternative plan—a principle that, with the exception of very small groups, holds true today. To reduce opposition from the medical community, a separate nonprofit health plan was set up to enroll members, and participating physicians organized their own independent medical group (now called the Permanente Medical Group) to contract with the Kaiser Foundation Health Plan.

Nixon Administration Promotes HMOs

Robert Kuttner (1998a, p. 1558) describes the transition from the founding principles of Kaiser Permanente to the initiatives of the Nixon administration and the subsequent development of HMOs: "The shift in prepaid group health care from an insurgent social movement to the most entrepreneurial and occasionally ruthless part of the health care system represents a stunning reversal. The turning point was in the early 1970s when President Nixon, 'rebaptized prepaid group health care plans as health maintenance organizations (HMOs), with legislation that provided for federal endorsement, certification, and assistance.'"

Ellwood's Proposal

In February 1970 Paul Ellwood, a Twin Cities physician and the founder of InterStudy (a highly respected source of information on the HMO industry), met with representatives of the Nixon administration to advocate ideas he had been promoting for several years. Starr (1982, p. 395) explains Ellwood's proposal: "The financing system, Ellwood argued, ought to reward health maintenance; prepayment for comprehensive care could achieve that end. So as an alternative to both fee-for-service and centralized governmental financing, Ellwood favored the development of comprehensive health care corporations, like the Kaiser plan. At a meeting in Washington, he first suggested calling them 'health maintenance organizations.'"

Nixon's Initiative

In February 1971 President Nixon announced a new national health strategy to control health care costs. The president pointed out that the health care system "operated episodically" on "illogical incentives," encouraging doctors to benefit from sickness rather than health. He said that HMOs reversed these incentives and called on Congress to establish planning grants and loan guarantees for the new HMOs. The administration's goal was to help create seventeen hundred HMOs by 1976, enrolling forty million people. There were thirty organizations that could be called HMOs in operation at the time this new program was announced. (See Starr, 1982, for a discussion of Nixon's health care initiative.)

HMO Act of 1973

The Nixon administration decided to push HMOs, and a 1973 law required businesses with twenty-five or more employees to offer at least one qualified HMO as an alternative to conventional insurance. This gave many of the newly established HMOs a significant marketing advantage; it was a door opener.

During this period it was mandatory for HMOs to use "community rating" in establishing monthly rates rather than the "experience rating" that became common in the mid-1980s (these two rating systems are discussed later in this chapter). Open enrollment regardless of health status was required for at least thirty days a year.

1976 to 1980: The HMO Steamroller Begins

The HMO program picked up momentum when Congress lifted several stringent requirements and reduced the mandatory benefits. "Then in May 1977, after seeing some routine data on federal employees showing that for every 1,000 people, Kaiser plan subscribers had only 349 days of hospitalization a year (compared to a national average of 1,149 days), Secretary Joseph Califano called for a review to see what needed to be done to revive federal HMO assistance. In 1978 Congress again amended the law to increase federal aid, and in that year HMO enrollment increased 1.4 million over the year before" (Starr, 1982, p. 415).

By mid-1979 there were 217 HMOs—about one-seventh the number the Nixon administration had anticipated. "Yet," as Starr (1982, p. 415) explains, "the total enrollment of 7.9 million people was twice as many as in 1970, and HMOs continued to perform well, providing medical care at significantly lower expense mainly because of reduced hospitalization."

HMO Growth over the Past Two Decades

Figure 2.2 shows the growth of HMOs by type (commercial, Medicare, and Medicaid) for the past twenty years. Exhibit 2.2 contains definitions of the various types of HMO. We estimate that by the end of 1999 HMO enrollment exceeded seventy-two million subscribers, including fifty-seven million covered under commercial policies.

Factors Driving HMO Growth

The rapid growth in HMO enrollment over most of the past twenty years is largely attributable to five factors:

Figure 2.2. HMO Enrollment by Type, 1980–2000.

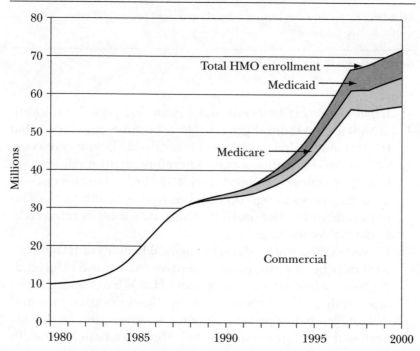

Sources: "Employer-Sponsored Health Plans," 1988; InterStudy,1997, pp. v–viii; authors' estimates.

Exhibit 2.2. Definitions of Five Types of HMO.

Staff model:	An HMO that delivers health services through a physician group that is employed by the HMO. PruCare was an example.
Group model:	An HMO that contracts with one independent group practice to provide health services. Kaiser Permanente is an example.
Network model:	An HMO that contracts with two or more independent group practices, possibly including a staff group, to provide health services. While a network may contain a few solo practices, it is predominantly organized around groups.
IPA model:	An HMO that contracts directly with physicians in independent practices; and/or contracts with one or more associations of physicians in independent practice; and/or contracts with one or more multi-specialty group practices.
Mixed model:	An HMO using a combination of the model types listed above.

Source: InterStudy, 1997, p. 113.

1. *Rapidly escalating health care costs.* Private and public employers, as well as the federal government, became convinced that HMOs could help control rapidly escalating health care costs, with no loss in quality of care. Therefore, many medium-sized to large employers offered the HMO alternative and encouraged employees to sign up with this type of health plan. (This requirement to offer an HMO alternative is often referred to as the "velvet hammer.")

2. *Comprehensiveness of benefits.* The medical benefits of HMOs have generally been more comprehensive than those offered by PPOs or traditional indemnity plans. HMOs have, for example, offered dental and vision coverage, lower copayments and deductibles, better prescription drug coverage, and more comprehensive wellness services. For Medicare beneficiaries in many metropolitan areas, enrolling in an HMO meant that they could drop their Medigap insurance. (Medigap insurance premiums have escalated rapidly over the past decade and typically exceed $200 per month per enrollee.)

3. *Lower PMPM rates.* HMO PMPM rates have consistently been 10 to 20 percent below the cost of traditional indemnity insurance, and a few percentage points below those charged by PPOs.

4. *Loosening of HMOs' restrictions.* Especially over the past five years HMOs have loosened their restrictions, most notably the need to go through a primary care gatekeeper, and have begun to allow subscribers to visit a favorite physician (either primary care or specialist) without large financial penalties. In other words most HMOs have responded to marketplace pressures for greater freedom of choice by offering POS plans.

5. *Satisfaction with HMOs.* Most employees and their dependents are satisfied with their HMO and have not been put off by highly publicized examples of denial of care or adverse publicity and jokes.

Issues for the Future of HMOs

What we have described so far in this chapter does not sound like an industry in retreat. However, despite the rapid growth and success of these types of health plans, HMOs carry significant baggage into the new millennium. Here are five challenges facing HMOs:

1. *Decline of HMOs' cost advantage.* The favorable cost advantage of HMOs has declined as other types of health plans and provider organizations have learned (usually from HMOs) how to do a better job of managing inpatient admissions.

2. *Limited opportunities for growth.* Because HMOs now constitute a mature industry, especially in the commercial sector, growth opportunities are limited. (There are still some states where HMO market penetration is relatively low, but these are generally not as heavily populated as the mature managed care markets.)

3. *Obstacles to expansion into the Medicare market.* There are serious problems and financial limitations to expanding into the Medicare market—one of the areas frequently identified as representing growth opportunities for most HMOs.

4. *Decreased competitive ability of smaller HMOs.* The benefits of economies of scale and increased clout with physicians and hospitals are substantial for larger health plans. This has led to

a large number of health plan consolidations (see Chapter Ten) and increased competition for smaller HMOs.

5. *Resistance on the part of physicians.* In many markets physicians are increasingly digging in their heels relative to capitation rates and the organization of delivery systems. Some physicians, for example, are establishing primary care networks and letting these groups contract with specialists. Negotiations with physician groups are becoming more rancorous. (Relations with physicians are discussed later in this chapter.)

PPOs Come on Strong in the Mid-1980s

From an employer and employee perspective PPOs have worked surprisingly well and have generally avoided the adverse media coverage of HMOs. We estimate that in 2000 there were one thousand PPOs in existence, with nearly seventy-five million Americans eligible to use the services of these health plans.

How PPOs Work

PPO customers have enjoyed one major advantage over HMO subscribers: when they receive treatment outside the preferred panel of physicians, they receive partial reimbursement, typically 80 to 90 percent of the allowed cost. This is referred to as "steering" patients to PPO providers by using financial incentives. By contrast, when subscribers to traditional HMOs go outside the authorized panel, they receive no financial benefits.

PPOs: An Interim Step?

Many human resources representatives in companies offering health plans thought of PPOs initially as a way to introduce employees to managed care and thus set the stage for the "normal" progression to HMOs. Experience with PPOs encouraged employees and their families to dip their toes into the cold water of managed care without being thrown into the icy river of more restrictive plans.

The broader panels of physicians and hospitals typical of PPOs make it difficult to control utilization. In PPOs physicians are paid on a discounted fee-for-service basis so the financial incentives are to increase volume rather than control utilization. Therefore, as a way for employers to control their health care costs, PPOs are suspect. This is an extremely important point when assessing the ability of managed care to limit the growth of health care spending (see Chapters Four and Five).

Physicians' Perspective on PPOs

For many physicians their first experience with managed care has been joining an IPA to contract with a PPO. The early PPOs promised access to more patients in return for discounts from physicians and hospitals. This of course turned out to be one of the empty promises of the managed care revolution. Physicians and hospitals ended up with most of the same patients and received less money for providing the same services.

Growth of PPOs

In 1980 PPOs were no more than a blip on the radar screen, but they came on strong beginning in the mid-1980s. By the late 1990s the number of PPO eligibles exceeded the number of persons covered under HMOs. By "eligibles" we mean the number of employees and their family members who are eligible to use the services of a PPO. Being eligible does not necessarily mean receiving care from a PPO. There is also some double counting because an employer may offer two or more PPOs and has no control over which of the PPOs employees and their families actually use. Despite these data limitations there can be no doubt that PPOs, the second half of the managed care spectrum, have experienced explosive growth and remain popular among employers and employees.

Issues for the Future of PPOs

These are five issues and opportunities that will likely shape the future of PPOs:

1. *Investment in infrastructure.* One of the issues for PPOs is investing in the infrastructure needed for success in the future, such as marketing, management, and administrative staff, IT, and medical management systems.

2. *Undercapitalization.* Our experience indicates that most PPOs are undercapitalized; network access fees do not provide sufficient capital. Because PPOs do not accept risk, many leaders of these organizations would argue that they do not need the same amount of capital required by HMOs. However, many PPOs are tremendously undercapitalized and skimp on building their infrastructure.

3. *Lack of primary care physicians.* Many PPOs contract with IPAs that are dominated by medical specialists and are weak in terms of their primary care physician base. In many instances the motivation of specialists to be part of a PPO is solely to maintain access to patients by being on as many provider panels as possible. In fact, we know of cases where specialists are members of more than thirty PPOs. As one surgeon told us, "Why not? It doesn't cost much to be in an IPA or contract with a PPO. And, there aren't that many requirements or hoops that we have to jump through. Sure, it is cumbersome to have so many different contracts, but that seems like a relatively small price to pay to continue to have access to my patients."

4. *Competitive advantage.* On the positive side PPOs and IPAs have proved to be nimble on their feet in competing for business and aggressively pricing contracts with employers. In some markets PPOs and their physicians are doing what it takes to maintain or improve their competitive position, including offering dramatic price concessions.

5. *Successful patient and hospitalization management.* Many PPOs have become adept at managing patients, particularly in keeping patients out of hospitals or reducing length of stay. Better management of hospitalization is probably the most important initiative for a PPO that wants to improve its competitive position relative to HMOs.

Managed Care in Government Programs

One of the major shifts in managed care over the past few years has been its use by federal and state governments in attempting to control costs in the Medicare and Medicaid programs.

Managed Care Comes to the Rescue of Medicare

An average 5 to 6 percent annual increase in Medicare spending between 1988 and 1996 prompted policymakers to look to the principles of managed care as a way to slow the rate of spending. The reasoning: It worked well in the private sector, so why would it not work for Medicare?

Health plans were slow to get into Medicare HMOs under the cost-based payment structure originally used by HCFA, but then several decided to pursue Medicare risk contracting. Under this type of risk arrangement health plans are typically paid 95 percent of the average adjusted per capita cost (AAPCC) of beneficiaries in a given county after adjustments for age, sex, and institutional status. In some metropolitan markets the AAPCC was sufficiently high—say $600 or more per month—to offer additional benefits to members to attract them to the health plan without losing money.

Savings in Medicare Risk Plans

A study by the AARP found that enrollees in Medicare risk plans spend one-third less than fee-for-service beneficiaries with private supplemental insurance (Walker, 1998). By shifting the risk to providers and exacting discounts for inpatient and other services, health plans offering Medicare risk plans benefited from lower medical costs compared with traditional fee-for-service arrangements that have no restriction on the choice of physicians or hospitals.

Growth in Enrollment

Enrollment in Medicare risk plans jumped from just about three million in 1995 to an estimated eight million in 2000. Major players like PacifiCare expanded eastward from California with aggressive marketing that earned them nearly one million Medicare subscribers by March 1999, or about 16 percent of all Medicare risk enrollees nationally. Kaiser Permanente is another health plan with a large base of Medicare recipients.

Medicare+Choice Program

With the movement of over 15 percent of the Medicare population into risk plans, Congress saw the opportunity to curb the program's rising expenditures by encouraging more beneficiaries to enroll in managed care plans. As part of the BBA of 1997, Congress created the Medicare+Choice program.

Much like the range of options that exist in the private market, Medicare+Choice established several choices for beneficiaries: HMOs, HMO POS plans, PPOs, PSOs that can essentially function like HMOs, medical savings accounts (MSAs), and traditional indemnity insurance. The BBA also reduced future Medicare expenditures by implementing a 2 percent cap on AAPCC increases for two years and leveling out some of the wide variation in AAPCC rates that existed around the country.

However, cutting back payment rates backfired, and the Medicare+Choice program has been slow to take off. In fact, citing inadequate payment, several large health plans, including Aetna U.S. Healthcare and United HealthCare, pulled out of a number of predominantly rural markets in 1998 and 1999. Although the net effect of these withdrawals affected a small percentage of all Medicare beneficiaries, the actions of these large plans drew severe criticism from HCFA officials and added more fuel to the fire of public backlash against managed care.

Medicaid Gets into Managed Care

In an effort to curb Medicaid expenditures, nearly every state has introduced some form of managed care. The number of Medicaid beneficiaries enrolled in managed care plans increased from 1.7 million in 1993 to 7.5 million in 2000. The percentage of Medicaid beneficiaries under managed care plans is highest in urban areas.

In some instances implementing managed care was as simple as requiring beneficiaries to select a primary care physician as the central coordinator of their care. In other cases states have contracted with health plans to care for the Medicaid population. These health plans in turn contract with providers (often on a risk basis) to provide medical care. Other states rely on community health clinics and other providers to assume responsibility for this population; these arrangements usually do not include the assumption of full financial risk.

It has been difficult for most states to find health plans ready and willing to serve the Medicaid population consistently. Many HMOs have withdrawn from the program or frozen their enrollment, thus impeding efforts to encourage more enrollment in managed care. In rural areas, where there are no managed care plans or providers are not under pressure to accept risk or discounted fee structures, there has been virtually no growth in Medicaid risk products.

Long-Term Care

Although managed care has penetrated the younger Medicaid population, it has not been applied to long-term care or disabled individuals. (Services to the disabled and elderly constitute about half of all Medicaid expenditures.) Instead Medicaid is attempting to shift reimbursement away from nursing homes to more home- and community-based providers, including assisted living, adult day programs, and in-home services.

Health Care Coverage Patterns: Summary

Table 2.1 shows our estimates of the access to health care coverage for the entire U.S. population. This includes the number of persons on Medicare (seniors and disabled) and Medicaid (both those in nursing homes and those receiving medical coverage), children on the Children's Health Insurance Program (CHIPS), employees and their families with health insurance coverage (85 percent in managed care), CHAMPUS (the program for dependents of military personnel), the self-insured, and the uninsured.

We estimate that the number of individuals with traditional indemnity coverage dropped from 94 million in 1990 to around 17 million in 2000—a decline of 77 million persons in ten years. The number of Medicare recipients increased to 40 million (most of whom have the equivalent of indemnity insurance—inasmuch as they have, for example, freedom of choice). Most important and of great concern, the number of the uninsured increased by

Table 2.1. Number of Americans by Type of Health Care Coverage, 1990, 1995, and 2000.

Type of Coverage	1990	1995	2000
Government			
Medicare—65+	27	32	35
Medicare—disabled	3	4	5
Medicaid—medical	27	33	31
Children's health insurance program	—	—	5
Subtotal	57	69	76
Uninsured	31	40	45
Subtotal	88	109	121
Employer			
HMOs (commercial only)	33	45	57
PPOs	29	45	67
Indemnity and other	94	55	17
Subtotal	156	145	141
Self-insurance	7	9	13
CHAMPUS, institutionalized	9	9	9
Total	260	272	284

Note: Figures represent millions.

14 million over the past decade—from 31 million in 1990 to 45 million in 2000. In aggregate the number of employees and their families covered by health insurance at work has declined over the same ten-year period from 156 million to 141 million.

On the positive side more than 75 percent of all employers offered health benefits to their employees in 1996, up from 72 percent in 1987. However, the percentage of employees who elected coverage through their employer declined from 88 percent in 1987 to 80 percent in 1996 (Kuttner, 1999). A Kaiser Family Foundation report conducted in conjunction with the Commonwealth Fund found that 80 percent of adults without health insurance coverage were employed or part of working families (Kaiser Family Foundation, 1999).

The AFL-CIO and the Lewin Group examined why fewer workers and their families are being covered by employer-based health insurance. Although expansion in Medicaid programs and lower earnings explain part of the story, the report found that in three-fourths of the cases rising employee premiums discouraged employees from accessing health care coverage through their employers (*Medical Benefits*, 1998).

Some consumers are opting not to take employer-sponsored coverage because of the cost; others are paying for it out of their disposable income. Research by the Consumers Union indicates that one out of eight families under retirement age spent more than 10 percent of its income on premiums and out-of-pocket health care costs in 1996—despite the fact that 80 percent of these families had health insurance for every family member (Shearer, 1998). The research also noted that moderate-income families (those with an income of $30,000 to $40,000 per year) paid $1,500 per year in health insurance premiums and out-of-pocket medical costs.

Regional Variations in Managed Care Coverage

Since its inception, the development and spread of managed care has been uneven. California, Oregon, Washington, Arizona, Massachusetts, and Minnesota have traditionally had higher HMO market penetration than most other states. Wisconsin, Michigan, Pennsylvania, Florida, and Colorado also have high levels of HMO coverage. The less populated states in the Upper Midwest and many in the Southeast have experienced little or no HMO market penetration. Physicians and hospitals in states like Montana are just entering the managed care revolution.

Why the differences? The contrast between the dominance of HMOs in some states and the relative absence of managed care in others has much to do with population density, size of multispecialty medical groups, and whether or not there is a large surplus of physicians. In heavily populated states with a surplus of physicians, employers and health plans have more market power and a greater ability to dictate how physicians will be paid.

Another interesting point in assessing HMO market penetration is that there are tremendous variations even within the markets most heavily saturated by managed care. In California, for example, the managed care penetration rates outside the major metropolitan areas often resemble those of Montana or Kansas. As just discussed, low population density and the ratio of physicians to population appear to be the determining factors.

Market Stages of Managed Care

There are a number of approaches for evaluating the status of managed care in a community or region. One model, used by VHA Inc. (1996), is based on four stages of managed care markets (summarized in Figure 2.3):

Stage I: Many rural areas are in Stage I, which is characterized by no limits, freedom of choice, viable solo practices, and the beginning of physician anxiety.

Stage II: In those parts of the country in Stage II, costs are beginning to matter, overcapacity of specialists and hospitals exists, purchasers have some market power, and physicians are "highly" anxious.

Stage III: For those few markets in Stage III the market defines price, excess capacity has been eliminated from payments (as in Southern California), and the market demands "real" managed care, not just discounts.

Stage IV: Stage IV resembles the Buyer's Health Care Action Group (BHCAG) initiative in the Twin Cities, where providers are accountable for quality, service, and access, incentives to do the "wrong thing" are eliminated, and purchasers—both employers and employees—have full market power.

It appeared for a time that managed care would develop according to these four stages, and to a limited extent it has. However, employers and Medicare have not been as demanding as originally anticipated; therefore in most markets managed care appears to be stalled in Stages II and III.

Community and Experience Rating

Managed care has been a major force in shifting health insurance coverage from "community rating" to "experience rating." In the

Figure 2.3. Four Market Stages of Managed Care.

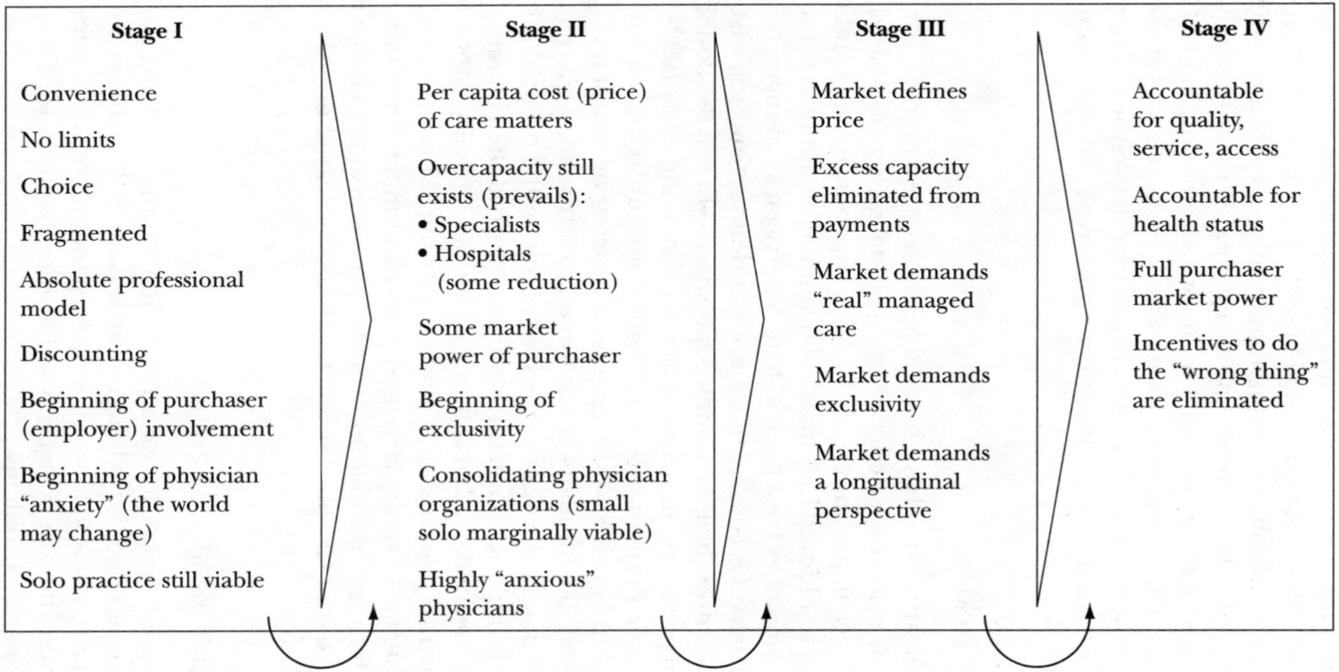

Stage I	Stage II	Stage III	Stage IV
Convenience	Per capita cost (price) of care matters	Market defines price	Accountable for quality, service, access
No limits	Overcapacity still exists (prevails):	Excess capacity eliminated from payments	Accountable for health status
Choice	• Specialists		
Fragmented	• Hospitals (some reduction)	Market demands "real" managed care	Full purchaser market power
Absolute professional model	Some market power of purchaser	Market demands exclusivity	Incentives to do the "wrong thing" are eliminated
Discounting	Beginning of exclusivity	Market demands a longitudinal perspective	
Beginning of purchaser (employer) involvement	Consolidating physician organizations (small solo marginally viable)		
Beginning of physician "anxiety" (the world may change)	Highly "anxious" physicians		
Solo practice still viable			

Source: VHA Inc., 1996, p. 23.

early to mid-1980s, when managed care began its big push, the statewide Blue Cross and Blue Shield systems, which often dominated their markets, used community rating—everyone in the community paid the same premium for health insurance coverage regardless of their physical condition. As one hospital CEO said, "This was true insurance. Those who were healthy paid the costs of the sick. Since health care costs were relatively low, and premiums not burdensome for most employers, no one seemed to object."

Cherry Picking

Many health plans have been able to carve out markets for themselves by using experience rating—rating each group based on its experience in previous years. By using experience rating and underpricing traditional indemnity plans, some health plans and insurance companies have been able to "cherry pick" younger, healthier subscribers. Of course, this has left indemnity and self-insurance plans to cover the less healthy populations—hence the double-digit annual premium increases of the late 1980s and early 1990s.

Kaiser Permanente stuck with community rating for many years, but because of the aggressive pricing of competing HMOs and other health plans, it was forced to introduce experience rating. Although this flies in the face of one of the original purposes of the founders, competitive pressures forced the change.

As the 1990s faded into history, it was virtually impossible to find health plans using community rating. This has been a contributing factor to the large and growing number of the uninsured. The Heritage Foundation proposal for a consumer choice model (discussed in Chapter Twelve) calls for increased use of community rating.

Impact of Mandated Coverage

Jeff Goldsmith argues for a return to community rating based on the strong possibility that genetic testing will enable consumers and health plans to more fully understand the risks of insuring certain individuals and that this will lead to a multitude of insurance underwriting problems.

"It makes sense," Goldsmith (1998b, p. 46) contends, "that at some point in this increasingly unforgiving political climate, insurers will find it advantageous to cut their losses, voluntarily end the conventional insurance underwriting process and embrace community rating of health and life insurance instead."

Goldsmith is concerned, however, that a return to community rating might have unintended consequences, such as an increasing number of younger workers opting out of their employer's health plan (because costs may go up) and joining the ranks of the uninsured. "Given the large discretionary component in individuals' decisions not to seek health coverage, it is highly unlikely that the U.S. will be able to achieve universal coverage without mandating that individuals purchase health insurance for themselves and their families" (Goldsmith, 1998b, p. 46). This mandate is part of the consumer choice model discussed in Chapter Twelve.

Anne Ladd, who has consulted on the start-up of two health insurance purchasing cooperatives and is now product manager for Micromedex, a medical database company, suggests that "adjusted community rating" would be the best option for a return to community rating. She told us:

> I agree with Goldsmith that pure community rating has the young, healthy male subsidizing the older, unhealthy person. The result is that the young and healthy opt out of the system. The best solution I have seen is adjusted community rating, where you create age bands—a pool of say eighteen- to twenty-five-year-olds, and another pool of twenty-five- to forty-year-olds, etc. In this way you don't price the young, healthy people out of the pool. Other logical adjustments to the community rating are sex and geography. Women in their childbearing years are more expensive to cover than young men, and the cost of medical care often varies along with the cost of living.

Physicians and Managed Care

There are differing views on the role of physicians and managed care. For example, there is little doubt that a majority of physicians are unhappy with managed care. Another view is that managed care has proved its value by controlling the rate of increase in health care costs and improving quality and that the next generation of physicians will not have to be sold on its value.

Physicians as a Problem for Managed Care

Thomas Bodenheimer, M.D., (1999, p. 584) reports that "nearly 70 percent of 6,000 physicians in 22 markets surveyed in 1998 characterized themselves as against managed care." Numerous other surveys in the mid- to late 1990s reached the same conclusion. Alain Enthoven, a professor at Stanford University, believes that physicians are "the main source of energy in the managed care backlash." He says, "Physicians are angry over their loss of authority, autonomy and income. They want more money and freedom to practice." He also says that from the viewpoint of physicians, managed care is "maddeningly complex" (Enthoven, 1998, p. 3). John Cochrane (1999a, p. 12), former editor of *Integrated Healthcare Report,* believes that physicians' underlying sources of irritation with managed care are loss of autonomy, interference with the patient care process, the number of hoops to jump through, and lack of a voice in the process.

Of course, UnitedHealth Group's decision to do away with pre-authorizations is likely to be the health plan industry's first step toward improving its relationship with physicians and its image with patients. Physicians will not have to defend their decisions on referrals or services provided. Princeton health economist Uwe Reinhardt comments, "Why did it take these guys 10 years to figure this out?" (Gentry, 1999b, p. B6).

Fee-for-Service Abuses Leading to Managed Care

Another view is that by their greed and unwillingness to come to grips with unexplained clinical variations, physicians (not all, but a sizable proportion) brought on the need for HMOs. One friend of the authors, a twenty-five-year veteran of managed care, said, "In many ways managed care saved employers and Medicare from bankruptcy. It may not have stopped the 'rape and pillage' by some medical practitioners, but at least managed care slowed down a lot of disgraceful behavior."

Without using terminology quite this strong, we admit to being bothered by the large amount of inappropriate and unnecessary medical care. The studies of Dr. John Wennberg and his colleagues at Dartmouth (Dartmouth Medical School, 1996) amply prove the continued existence of a high degree of clinical variation (and this variation has been going on for decades) that is cause for concern.

Is Managed Care Meeting Its Original Objectives?

How well have managed care plans met their dual objectives of reducing health care costs and improving the overall health status of their members (or "covered lives" in HMO parlance)?

Reducing Costs

Managed care has helped lower the annual rate of growth in the portion of health care costs borne by employers. For the 1993 through 1997 period, the rate of increase in medical costs only slightly exceeded that of the consumer price index (CPI). (See Figure 2.4.) This compares with double-digit gains in health care costs (and revenues for providers) that far outstripped increases in the CPI during most of the 1980s, before managed care had significant market share.

But managed care should not be given all the credit. As shown in Figure 2.4, general price inflation was low in the 1990s, and this helped hold down the overall rate of increase in health care costs. In addition, Medicare was a generous payer during most of the 1990s (until 1998, when the provisions of the BBA began to kick in). This took cost-shifting pressures off employers and their managed care intermediaries. Our analysis indicates that during the 1990s Medicare recipients moved from being subsidized by employers and individuals to paying more than their full share of costs, thus bearing some of the burden of financial shortfalls from those on Medicaid and the uninsured (we address this issue in detail in Chapter Five).

Managed Care's Impact on Quality

On the quality issue representatives of major employers (including the Washington Business Group on Health) and health plans

**Figure 2.4. Average Change in the Consumer Price Index
and Medical Care Costs, 1980–2000.**

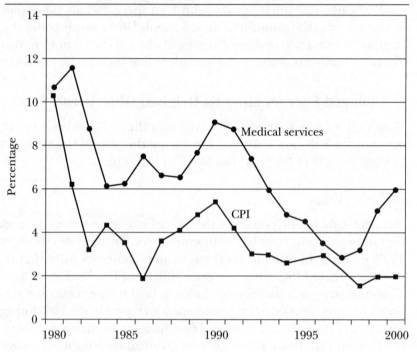

Sources: U.S. Department of Labor; authors' estimates.

(including Kaiser Permanente) were instrumental in establishing
the National Council on Quality Assurance (NCQA) and the
Health Plan Employer Data and Information Set (HEDIS) measures of quality. The founders of these quality measures argue that
many managed care plans have had a positive impact on quality.
The NCQA credentialing process and annual "report cards" support this finding.

Anecdotal experience appears to reign over hard data. Those
patients and families who report bad experiences with managed
care plans are unlikely to be persuaded by NCQA accreditation or
the monitoring of how well plans meet the HEDIS guidelines. They
are often concerned about the lack of choice of physicians and by
what they perceive as the withholding of medical services, such as
bone marrow transplants, in acute cases.

The science of quality measurement in health care remains in its infancy. Despite much discussion about measuring and reporting on quality, much remains to be done. Most efforts to measure quality include surveys of patients regarding their satisfaction with recent visits to a physician or hospital and broad measures of the health status of the population (for example, percentage of women over forty who have had mammograms in the past two years or the proportion of men tested for prostate cancer). We anticipate major gains in the ability of health care providers and health plans to measure quality of care, especially with the growth of electronic medical records and enterprise databases (discussed in Chapter Eight).

Financial Incentives and Quality

Acknowledging that most physicians abhor HMOs and capitation (some refer to capitation as "obscene"), Emily Friedman (1998, p. 8), a health care ethicist, points out that all financial incentives, including fee-for-service arrangements, involve moral hazards: "What is ethically superior about an incentive—the dominant one in healthcare until a few years ago—that encourages physicians to do every possible test, order every possible image, and even perform surgery or other procedures that are only marginally necessary (if that) simply because if you don't do them, you don't get paid?"

We agree with Friedman's argument: capitation and managed care, by themselves, are not inferior in terms of the quality of care delivered under these financial arrangements. It is difficult to find data that sustain the argument that managed care has a negative impact on quality or to support the hypothesis that fee-for-service leads to higher quality.

Value Added: More Than Quality and Costs

Part of the problem in evaluating managed care is that we may not be asking the right questions or considering the right measures. The key is value added, a broader concept that includes more than clinical quality and annual increases in costs. Value added includes service, convenience, access, relationships with physicians, innovation, unit prices, and the volume or intensity of use of certain resources (for example, number of inpatient days per thousand members).

Regarding whether managed care is meeting its objectives, we have already said that it has had a favorable impact in terms of reducing the annual increase in employer and employee health care costs—both prices and volume of services. As noted previously, the best managed care plans are able to provide evidence that they are offering high-quality care, reducing inpatient hospitalizations, and cutting the amount of clinical variation. In our view most of the problems with managed care relate to adverse publicity over denial of certain medical procedures, access, service, and relationships with personal physicians. Many managed care plans would not score well in these important areas of value added.

Conclusions

Robert Kuttner (1998a, p. 1562) describes the double paradox that consumers, employers, and managed care companies face: "The more patients chafe under the constraints of utilization controls, the more they demand a choice of doctors—not realizing that the various doctors affiliated with a plan have similar or identical financial incentives to constrain costs. And the more plans try to offer a choice, the further they stray from the systemwide integration, prevention, and case management that are the supposed advantages of HMOs." This double paradox is one of the many weaknesses of managed care. Another paradox is that the media highlight managed care plans (usually HMOs) for alleged abuses or withholding expensive treatments, while at the same time a continuing stream of surveys show high levels of member satisfaction and the efforts of NCQA result in the accreditation of many HMOs.

To focus on the denial of medical services and the overall thrust of many managed care plans to reduce the quantity of health care services consumed is to focus on only half of the story. Consider Wennberg's studies, compiled over the past twenty years, showing the continued existence of large, unexplained variations in utilization of medical services. Female residents of one community having three times the number of hysterectomies as those in a neighboring community with the same demographic characteristics would be an example of such variation. Although there is little disagreement that health care is local, we believe that these very significant variations indicate poor quality of care. Because many physicians are solidified in their opposition to managed care, they need to be more forthright in discussing possible reasons for these variations. The evidence suggests that part of the reason is the availability (or surplus) of certain specialists in the communities being compared.

What can we learn from this summary of the origins and growth of HMOs and PPOs and their dominant position as the organizations financing a very large portion of health care? Here are several observations:

The founding principles of managed care are still relevant today. The principles articulated by Henry Kaiser and the goals of Congress and the Nixon administration in the 1970s appear to be as relevant today as when they were first articulated. The emphasis on prevention, early detection of diseases, and coordinated care for those who are sick is as timely today as in the 1930s on the Colorado River aqueduct.

The financial strains facing managed care have not changed much. Questionable prospects for economic viability faced Henry Kaiser, Sidney Garfield, and others in deciding whether the Kaiser plan should stay in business beyond the end of World War II. Even though it was created as a not-for-profit organization, there was concern about whether Kaiser Permanente could compete and stay afloat financially. These same issues of financial performance dog HMOs today, with special pressure on those that are publicly owned with shares traded on Wall Street.

Capitation as a payment mechanism appears to have peaked. This raises serious questions about the future of HMOs and the concept of shifting risk and accountability to physicians and hospitals. Furthermore, it leaves health care's financial incentives in disarray. Hopefully IT, clinical guidelines, and better outcomes measurement systems will offer part of the answer. (Shifting risk to physicians through capitation is discussed in Chapter Twelve.)

Genetic research and new drugs have the potential to substantially alter health care financing. What can we expect from genetic research and new drugs in terms of negative impact on the finances of managed care plans? The original HMOs provided comprehensive medical services, including prescription drug coverage. However, with the rapid escalation in the number and price of popular new drugs, the objective of providing members with prescription drugs at low copayments may no longer be achievable without major changes in the structure of health plans.

Consumer empowerment and choice increase the pressure for change. Can managed care adapt to the developing movement toward consumer empowerment and choice? Or to the declining role of employers as providers of health care coverage and the need for consumers to take more responsibility for their own health? We believe that managed care can adapt and survive under these circumstances but not without profound changes.

Managed care must reclaim the support of consumers and providers. How can managed care, and HMOs in particular, regain public trust and support from physicians? UnitedHealth's decision to end prospective review was one step in the right direction.

Managed care is a mature industry. Without a substantial boost in enrollment in Medicare+Choice, managed care is fully developed. The double-digit annual increases in covered lives are a thing of the past. As with most mature industries, we can expect to see more price competition (which means more pressure on physicians and hospitals). The rate increases managed care firms have sought from the late 1990s and into the twenty-first century are probably not sustainable, especially in scenarios 1 and 2 (see Chapter Thirteen).

We address these and related questions about the future of managed care in subsequent chapters. We now turn our attention to the overall size, shape, and dynamics of the health care marketplace of the future.

Financial Resources Available to Fund Health Care

The health care marketplace is huge. At $1.3 trillion and growing at about $100 billion per year, you can't tell me that there isn't enough money to go around.

RADIOLOGIST, DENVER

The health care market in the United States is disproportionately large compared with that of other developed countries—35 percent larger than Canada's as a percentage of GDP and more than twice as large as in most other countries. The three chapters making up Part Two focus on the size and dynamics of the U.S. health care marketplace, the forces driving health care spending, and the direction in which the market is headed in the new millennium. In Part Two we also discuss who is buying health care services at full cost or more and who is receiving discounts or paying nothing.

In Chapter Three we discuss the various elements of health care in terms of who is paying—Medicare, Medicaid, employers, and individuals—and the rates of growth of each element of the payer mix. Chapter Three also includes an analysis of where health care dollars are being spent and how this has changed over the past two decades.

Direction of the Health Care Market over the Next Five Years

Chapter Four includes our analysis of the forces that have driven health care spending (or costs to payers) over the past decade. This forms the basis for projecting future health care spending, or the growth in the overall health care marketplace, in the years ahead. Most of the forces driving health care costs in the United States are expected to continue to move costs upward. This suggests significant increases in health care spending in the future. We project that the overall market will reach $1.8 trillion by 2005 in our incremental-change scenario (scenario 1). It will be even higher in scenario 3, where technology dominates.

Who Pays for and Who Receives Medical Services

Over the past two decades there have been fundamental changes in who is paying for health care versus who is receiving the benefits. The discontinuities in terms of who pays and who receives medical services is a continuing source of instability for the U.S. health care system.

It was common knowledge ten to twelve years ago that private indemnity insurance (mostly provided by employers) was subsidizing Medicare, Medicaid, and the uninsured. Then along came managed care, with its discounts and lower payments, replacing indemnity insurance and making Medicare the preferred payer of many physicians and hospitals.

With the number of the uninsured continuing to increase and Medicare ratcheting down its payment levels, will managed care be able to keep employers' health care spending down? We do not believe that managed care as presently structured will be able to limit employers' spending. Therefore we anticipate radical changes in managed care with respect to its structure, financial incentives, use of information systems, and relationships with providers.

The Uninsured

At the end of the twentieth century the uninsured numbered close to forty-five million, or about 17 percent of the country's population.

Most physicians and hospital administrators argue that despite their inability (or unwillingness) to pay, these individuals receive health care services, often in the hospital or in emergency situations.

Medicare

Medicare has emerged as the largest and most rapidly growing purchaser of health care services. By the end of the 1990s Medicare, combined with Medicaid and other state and federal programs, accounted for 35 percent of all health care spending in the United States. Will the BBA be successful in reducing the rate of increase in Medicare spending, or will HCFA be compelled to continue to pay its fair share of health care costs? This is a crucial question for most hospitals and medical specialists.

Consumers

A less subtle change has been the shift toward consumers paying an increasing share of their health care costs. Some of this has been involuntary—employers have insisted on higher copayments and deductibles and on employees paying a bigger share of insurance premiums. At the same time the growth in voluntary consumer spending for many health care products and services has been staggering. This includes cosmetic surgery, in vitro fertilization, laser eye surgery, alternative medicines and therapies, glasses and contact lenses, hearing aids, and the like.

Inequities in the Health Care System

We are also concerned about the fairness of the present system of shifting costs from the uninsured and Medicaid to employers and consumers. If Medicare is able to reduce the rate of increase in its spending, this will put even more pressure on managed care and its backers—the employers.

Our conclusion is that the federal government and consumers will become bigger and bigger players in the health care marketplace of the future. If we are correct, this shift has important long-term implications for physicians, hospitals, drug companies, other health care providers, and health plans.

Chapter Three

The Dynamics of the Health Care Marketplace

With the BBA and continued pressure from managed care,
I can understand why physicians and hospital managers
are depressed. However, the health care market is
increasingly dynamic, and future growth opportunities are
mind-boggling. It's an exciting time to be in health care.
HEALTH SYSTEM CEO

Viewed from any perspective, the U.S. health care industry is gigantic. In 2000 it accounted for $1.3 trillion in spending. Per capita health care spending in the United States was twice as high as in most other developed countries in the world. This chapter examines the historical growth, size, and shape of the U.S. health care marketplace from a number of different viewpoints and addresses the following questions:

- How big is the U.S. health care market? How much has it grown over the past two decades?
- What is the health care payer mix (the distribution of costs among Medicare, Medicaid, employers, consumers, and the uninsured) and how has it changed over the past twenty years?
- What share of health care spending goes to physicians, hospitals, pharmaceutical companies, nursing homes, and other providers? How has this changed over the past two decades?
- How much is spent on health care services for each major market segment: seniors, Medicaid, employers and employees, the self-insured, CHAMPUS, the uninsured, and others?

- What accounts for the differences between overall health care spending and the health plan premiums that employers pay?

Size and Growth of the Health Care Market

Exhibit 3.1 summarizes trends in health care spending between 1980 and 2000.

Health care spending in the United States has grown from $247 billion in 1980 to $1.3 trillion in 2000—up over 400 percent in twenty years (see Figure 3.1). These revenue increases equal a growth in health care's share of GDP from 8.9 percent in 1980 to 14.0 percent in 2000.

Whether viewed on a per capita basis or as a percentage of GDP, health care spending in the United States continues to be substantially higher than in any other developed country. John Iglehart (1999a) offers an explanation for the variation in health care spending between the United States and other countries. In the United States, says Iglehart, physicians are paid more, a day in

Exhibit 3.1. Highlights in the Growth of Health Care, 1980–2000.

- Health care spending in the United States—estimated at $1.3 trillion in 2000—has grown over 400 percent in two decades and accounts for 14 percent of GDP.
- U.S. health care spending is substantially higher than in any other developed country.
- The combination of Medicare and Medicaid increased from 25 percent of all health care dollars in 1980 to 34 percent in 2000.
- Hospitals' share of health care revenues dropped from 41.5 percent in 1980 to 32.5 percent in 2000.
- Health care spending on seniors and the disabled in 2000 represented 39.5 percent of all health care dollars; this is for 14.1 percent of the population.
- Between 1995 and 1998 the rate of increase in health care costs substantially exceeded health plan premium increases charged to employers.
- The sectors of health care showing the most growth in recent years have been drugs, nursing home care, home health, and other services (for example, personal care, administration).

Figure 3.1. National Health Expenditures in the United States, Actual and Inflation Adjusted, 1980–2000.

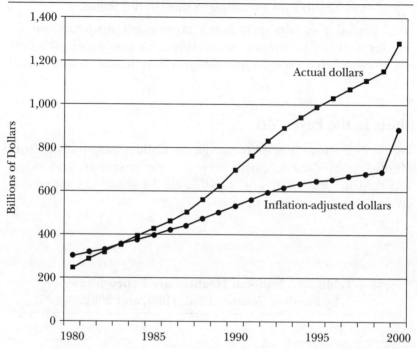

Sources: Health Care Financing Administration; Bureau of the Census; authors' estimates.

the hospital is considerably more expensive, and medical technology diffuses more rapidly and is used to treat more patients. In addition to these reasons, we propose five other factors that contribute to the disproportionately large U.S. health care market:

1. The competitive, free-market system in the United States lacks overall controls such as global budgeting.
2. High administrative overhead associated with the pluralistic, complex, and managed care–dominated U.S. system adds costs to health care.
3. Consumer demand for health care services is insatiable. Almost all physicians will agree that the "unrealistic expectations" of consumers are a key factor driving demand.

4. A surplus of medical specialists (such as orthopedic surgeons, anesthesiologists, radiologists, cardiologists, and urologists) adds to health care spending in the United States.

5. A period of sustained economic growth and prosperity and the desire of many employers to provide fairly generous health benefits lead to increased spending on health care in the United States.

Shifts in the Payer Mix

Figure 3.2 shows the percentage of dollars originating from Medicare, Medicaid, employers, private payment, and other sources for 1980, 1990, and 2000. Table 3.1 shows the actual dollar amounts for these same years.

Table 3.1. National Health Care Expenditures by Funding Source, 1980, 1990, and 2000.

Source of Funds	1980	1990	2000
Private funds			
Out-of-pocket payments	$ 60.3	$145.0	$207.2
Private health insurance	69.8	239.6	439.0
Other private funds	12.5	31.6	53.6
Subtotal	$142.5	$416.2	$699.8
Public funds			
Medicare	$ 37.5	$111.5	$255.5
Medicaid (federal and state)	26.1	75.4	190.7
Other federal	19.9	41.0	67.0
Other state and local	21.2	55.3	92.0
Subtotal	$104.8	$283.2	$605.2
Total	$247.3	$699.4	$1,305.0

Note: Figures represent billions.
Sources: Health Care Financing Administration; authors' estimates for 2000.

Figure 3.2. Distribution of National Health Care Funding Sources, 1980, 1990, and 2000.

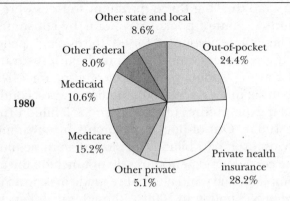

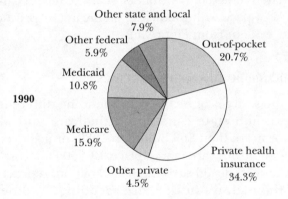

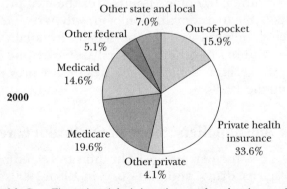

Sources: Health Care Financing Administration; authors' estimates for 2000.

Health Care Spending in 1980 and 2000

Twenty years ago the "big three" payment sources were private health insurance, out-of-pocket payments by consumers, and Medicare. These three accounted for two-thirds of all spending. By the end of the twentieth century private health insurance had moved into a strong leading position, accounting for $439 billion (up more than six times since 1980). Medicare was second in line, with estimated expenditures of more than $255 billion (up seven times since 1980). Out-of-pocket payments by consumers had increased to just over $207 billion (up more than three times since 1980). These consumer expenditures do not include the amounts spent on complementary and alternative medicines, which we estimate exceeded $53 billion in 2000. Although the dollars spent by consumers have increased, consumers' share of health care spending has not kept pace with Medicare, Medicaid, or private health insurance, as evident from Figure 3.2.

Medicare and Medicaid's Share Increases

Looking at the sources of health care spending differently, combined federal and state funding of Medicare and Medicaid accounted for more than $63 billion in 1980, or just over 25 percent of the total health care marketplace. By 2000 the combination of Medicare and Medicaid surpassed $446 billion, representing 34 percent of the nation's health care spending. In other words Medicare and Medicaid's share of health care spending has increased by nine percentage points over the past two decades. This has been due to a combination of growth in recipients of the two programs and improved reimbursement for Medicare. As we discuss in a number of other chapters, Medicare and Medicaid have been strong "growth markets" for health care providers, especially during the 1990s.

Providers' and Suppliers' Share of the Health Care Market

Figure 3.3 shows the percentage of health care spending for hospitals, physicians, drugs, and other uses in 1980, 1990, and 2000. Table 3.2 shows the actual dollar amounts for these same years.

Figure 3.3. Distribution of National Health Care Spending on Various Services, 1980, 1990, and 2000.

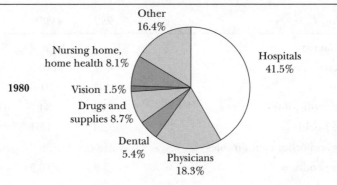

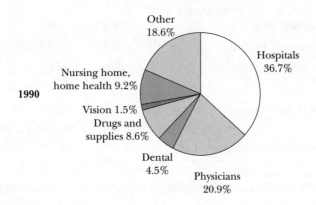

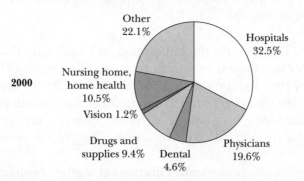

Sources: Health Care Financing Administration; authors' estimates for 2000.

Table 3.2. National Health Care Expenditure by Spending Category and GDP, 1980, 1990, and 2000.

Spending Category	1980	1990	2000
Hospital care	$102.7	$256.4	$ 422.8
Physician services	45.2	146.3	255.4
Dental	13.3	31.6	60.0
Other professional services	6.4	34.7	78.0
Home health	2.4	13.1	39.0
Drugs and other nondurables	21.6	59.9	122.3
Vision products	3.8	10.5	16.0
Nursing home care	17.6	50.9	97.0
Other personal care	4.0	11.2	40.0
Program administration and net cost of private health insurance	11.9	40.5	87.0
Government public health	6.7	19.6	47.0
Research and construction	11.6	24.5	36.0
Total	$247.3	$699.4	$1,300.5
Prescription drugs only	$ 12.0	$ 37.7	$ 90.0
GDP	$2,784	$5,744	$9,300
Total health care expenditures ÷ GDP	8.9%	12.2%	13.5%

Note: Figures represent billions.
Sources: Health Care Financing Administration; authors' estimates for 2000.

Here is how the major provider and supplier segments performed over the twenty-year period:

- *Hospitals.* Traditionally the largest user of health care dollars, hospitals experienced growth in revenues from nearly $103 billion in 1980 to an estimated $423 billion by 2000. However, even with dramatic growth in outpatient revenues (discussed in Chapter One), hospitals' share of total health care spending *dropped* from just 41.5 percent in 1980 to 32.5 percent in 2000.
- *Physicians and medical groups.* This market segment generated revenues of approximately $45 billion in 1980. By 2000

physicians' and medical groups' share of health care spending totaled over $255 billion. This represents a slight increase in market share, from 18.3 percent of all health care revenues in 1980 to 19.6 percent in 2000.

- *Drugs.* Pharmaceuticals have been the sleeper in driving health care revenues. In 1980 total spending on drugs was $12 billion; by 2000 the amount was $90 billion—a sevenfold increase. On a percentage basis the share of health care dollars spent on drugs has grown from just under 5 percent in 1980 to over 7 percent in 2000.

The remaining components of health care spending—vision, dental, home health, nursing homes, and other expenses—have grown from a combined $78 billion in 1980 to $525 billion in 2000. These items accounted for 35 percent of national health care spending in 1980. By 2000, however, these other components had increased in relative importance to 41 percent. Nursing home care, which rose from nearly $18 billion in 1980 to $97 billion by 2000, has been a major part of the growth in market share of these other items.

Estimates of Dollars Spent By Different Groups

The published statistics do not tell the whole story of spending patterns. Table 3.3 shows our estimates of the total dollars spent in 1980 through 2000 by or for seniors, younger persons on Medicaid, employees and their families, the self-insured, and the uninsured. Table 3.4 summarizes our estimates of the number of Americans in each segment of the health care marketplace and the share of the health care budget they spend.

Seniors and the Disabled

This group accounted for over $300 billion in spending in 1990 and $513 billion in 2000. This means that in 2000 health care spending for this population—a combination of Medicare, Medicaid, and private payment—was close to 40 percent of all health care costs. Seniors and the disabled represented just over 14 percent of the population in 2000.

**Table 3.3. Estimates of Health Care Spending
by Group, 1980, 1990, and 2000.**

	1980		1990		2000	
Source of Funds	Billions	Percent	Billions	Percent	Billions	Percent
Seniors and disabled (including nursing home)	$107.0	43.3	$304.0	43.5	$513.0	39.5
Medicaid (excluding nursing home)	8.5	3.5	24.5	3.5	97.3	7.5
CHIPS	—	—	—	—	3.0	0.2
Subtotal	$115.5	46.8	$328.5	47.0	$613.3	47.2
Employees and family members	$119.5	48.4	$339.5	48.6	$609.7	46.9
Self-insured	4.0	1.6	12.0	1.7	30.0	2.3
CHAMPUS, institutionalized	4.0	1.6	11.0	1.6	22.0	1.7
Subtotal	$127.5	51.6	$362.5	51.9	$650.7	50.1
Uninsured	$ 4.0	1.6	$ 8.0	1.1	$ 25.0	1.9
Total	$247.0	100.0	$699.0	100.0	$1,300.0	100.0

Source: Authors' estimates based on various sources, including Health Care Financing Administration; U.S. Department of Health and Human Services, 1998; Carrasquillo, Himmelstein, Woolhandler, and Bor, 1999; Kaiser Family Foundation, 1999; "Employer-Sponsored Health Plans," 1998; InterStudy, 1997; and Kuttner, 1999.

Although not indicated in Table 3.3, a subgroup of Medicare and Medicaid beneficiaries accounts for a disproportionate share of spending. Following the pattern of the past twenty years, 60 percent of Medicare's payments for the elderly and disabled are on behalf of 10 percent of enrollees. Dual-eligible beneficiaries (mostly in nursing homes)—about six million persons, representing just over 2 percent of the U.S. population—account for 30 percent of all Medicare spending and 35 percent of Medicaid spending (U.S. Department of Health and Human Services, 1998).

Table 3.4. Estimates of Population Size Versus Health Care Spending by Group, 2000.

	Number of People		Spending	
Source of Funds	Millions	Percent	Billions	Percent
Seniors and disabled	40	14.1	$513	39.5
Medicaid (excluding nursing home)	31	10.9	97	7.5
CHIPS	5	1.8	3	0.2
Uninsured, institutionalized	45	15.8	25	1.9
Employees and family members	141	49.6	610	46.9
Self-insured	13	4.6	30	2.3
CHAMPUS	9	3.2	22	1.7
Total	284	100.0	$1,300	100.0

Source: Authors' estimates based on various sources, including Health Care Financing Administration; U.S. Department of Health and Human Services, 1998; Carrasquillo, Himmelstein, Woolhandler, and Bor, 1999; Kaiser Family Foundation, 1999; "Employer-Sponsored Health Plans," 1998; InterStudy, 1997; and Kuttner, 1999.

Medicaid Recipients Not in Nursing Homes

In 1990 there were an estimated twenty-seven million individuals in this group; by 2000 thirty-one million were eligible to receive medical services through Medicaid. Medicaid spending for the younger participants has increased dramatically, from over $24 billion in 1990 to more than $97 billion in 2000. In 2000 Medicaid services (excluding nursing homes) absorbed 7.5 percent of all health care dollars on behalf of approximately 11 percent of the population. The estimated average per capita amount of health care dollars spent for those on Medicaid was $3,100 in 2000.

Employees and Their Families

Although the numbers have been declining over the past ten years, this is by far the largest group of Americans. The number of dollars spent by employers to provide health care for this group has increased from $240 billion in 1990 to $439 billion in 2000. When copayments, deductibles, and discretionary health care spending are added, employees and their families used more than $600 billion in health care services in 2000. This represented 46.9 percent of all health care spending, for the benefit of 141 million individuals—half of the U.S. population.

The Self-Insured

The number of people who are self-insured is estimated at thirteen million. Our estimate of the number of dollars associated with the self-insured population in 2000 is $30 billion. The spending of the self-insured represents 2.3 percent of the total health care budget.

The Uninsured

Numbering forty-five million in 2000, this group has increased by 50 percent over the past decade. We estimate that the uninsured pay for no more than a quarter of the cost of the health care resources they consume. Because they often do not access the health care system appropriately (less frequently, for example, through appointments with primary care or other physicians and more frequently through hospital emergency room visits), this is an expensive group to serve. The uninsured paid for an estimated $25 billion in health care services in 2000, or 1.9 percent of the total. The uninsured represented 15.8 percent of the population.

Reasons for the Variance Between Overall Health Care Spending and Health Plan Premiums

Explaining the variance between increases in premiums paid to health plans and increases in actual revenue to providers is one of the most complex aspects of health care economics. Employers and others often use the two measures interchangeably, and this is understandable. For most employers and employees the premiums they pay are their health care costs.

Between 1995 and 1998 premium increases did not keep pace with the growth in actual health care expenditures, and the medical loss ratio for HMOs (due to expenditures on physicians, hospitals, drugs, and other products and services) climbed to unacceptable levels. But in 1998 and 1999 most health plans pumped up their premiums—7.5 percent per year was the average—in an attempt to catch up with medical losses and regain profitability (Shinkman, 1999).

Underwriting Cycle

Many in the health plan industry have faith in the six-year underwriting cycle and its impact on the earnings of health plans. Based on the experience of the past twenty years, it would be difficult to argue against the existence of this cycle. Health plan profitability was strong in the early 1990s before taking a dip in the mid-1990s. The latest slump in profits lasted about three years. If the theory of the six-year cycle is correct, 1999 through 2001 will be years of higher premiums and improved profits for health plans.

Administrative Expenses and Medical Loss Ratios

Administrative expenses (including advertising and marketing) and medical loss ratios are the two cost factors that must be controlled if health plans are to achieve financial success. One approach to increasing market share is to lower prices, and many health plans elected to compete in this way in the mid-1990s. However, this has had the effect of increasing the medical loss ratios for most plans. In good times this ratio normally does not exceed 80 percent of health plan revenues. However, in 1997 and 1998, because of price competition, medical loss ratios of 85 to 95 percent or more were common. This example shows that even when annual increases in costs are reasonable, if health plan premiums are not raised as fast as or faster than the growth in actual health care costs, medical loss ratios will increase. Administrative expenses are the second major cost category for health plans. For a typical health plan administrative expenses—the cost of operating the infrastructure—would approximate 15 percent of revenues. Well-managed plans are able to get this ratio down to 12 percent.

Why Health Plan Premiums and Health Care Expenditures Do Not Correlate

It is apparent that the decision of many health plans to increase market share via price competition has been the major reason for the difference between increases in premiums and increases in actual health care costs during the period from 1995 through 1998. The health insurance six-year underwriting cycle is one way of explaining the divergences. In our view, however, the three years of profitable operation in the period from 1992 through 1995, followed by mounting losses in 1996 through 1998, were a reflection of the deliberate pricing and competitive strategies of many health plans.

Conclusions

At the close of the 1990s annual health care spending in the United States approached $1.3 trillion. Employers, Medicare, Medicaid, and the out-of-pocket payments of individuals accounted for more than 80 percent of dollars spent on health care. Consumers' share of spending (out-of-pocket payments) declined during most of the past two decades—dropping from 24.4 percent in 1980 to 15.9 percent in 2000—but turned around and began to grow more rapidly in the three years leading up to 2000.

The sectors of health care showing the largest percentage of growth over the past few years have been drugs, nursing homes and home health, and other services (personal care, program administration, and other professional services). The share of health care spending on hospitals has decreased substantially, from 41.5 percent in 1980 to 32.5 percent in 2000. Physicians' share of health care expenditures has increased slightly to almost 20 percent.

Seniors and the disabled accounted for about 14 percent of the population but consumed nearly 40 percent of all health care dollars. The uninsured represented almost 16 percent of the population but paid less than 3 percent of all health care costs.

In Chapter Four we will examine the various factors driving year-to-year increases in health care spending and discuss where health care expenditures are headed in the first five years of the twenty-first century.

How Health Care Spending Will Develop

Trends from 2000 to 2005

A seller's market for health care has been transformed into a buyer's market, the shape and direction of which remains cloudy and ill defined.

J. DANIEL BECKHAM, "The Obsolescence of Independent Practice," *Health Forum Journal,* March 1999

Our objective in this chapter is to offer insights about the future of a market that is "cloudy and ill defined." We consider two questions important to understanding where the health care marketplace is headed in the twenty-first century: What factors are most important in terms of their impact on health care spending? Where is health care spending, including health plan premiums paid by employers, headed in the years 2000–2005? Exhibit 4.1 summarizes expected trends in health care spending for the years 2000–2005.

Where Is Health Care Spending Headed?

We expect health care spending to increase by around 7 percent per year for the first five years of the twenty-first century. This is based on the incremental-change scenario (explained in detail in Chapter Thirteen). As we discuss in the paragraphs that follow, those factors weighing in on the side of increased expenditures far

Exhibit 4.1. Highlights in the Growth of
Health Care, 2000–2005.

- Health care spending will increase by $100 billion a year to $1.8 trillion by 2005. This is a substantially higher rate of increase than in the 1990s.
- Prescription drug spending is expected to increase from $90 billion in 2000 to $151 billion by 2005.
- Hospitals' share of the health care dollar will drop below 30 percent by 2005.
- Our analysis of the factors driving health care spending indicates that the most important are

    Increasing consumer expectations

    New drugs

    Medical and information technology

    Aging of the population

    Administrative expenses

    Surplus of physicians

---

exceed opportunities for payers to resist cost increases of this magnitude. By 2005 U.S. health care spending is expected to reach $1.8 trillion, approximately 15 percent of GDP. This would make health care a truly immense market for physicians, hospitals, and other providers of health-related goods and services.

Health Care Expenditures by Payer Category

Table 4.1 shows expected health care spending in 2005 by payer source. For example, Medicare is expected to reach $361 billion, up 41 percent over 2000 levels. Combined federal and state Medicaid spending can be expected to reach more than $286 billion, a 50 percent increase in five years. Out-of-pocket payments by consumers should increase by 32 percent.

Health Care Expenditures by Spending Category

Table 4.2 includes estimates of health care dollars likely to be spent on hospitals, physicians, and other providers.

Figure 4.1 depicts much of the same information in graphic form. According to the estimates shown in Figure 4.1, hospitals'

Table 4.1. National Health Care Expenditures
by Funding Source, 1995, 2000, and 2005.

Source of Funds	1995	2000	2005
Private funds			
Out-of-pocket payments	$171.0	$207.2	$272.7
Private health insurance	324.3	439.0	641.5
Other private funds	43.2	53.6	74.1
Subtotal	$538.5	$699.8	$988.3
Public funds			
Medicare	$185.2	$255.5	$361.0
Medicaid (federal and state)	146.1	190.7	286.2
Other federal	54.4	67.0	85.5
Other state and local	69.5	92.0	122.0
Subtotal	$455.2	$605.2	$854.7
Total	$993.7	$1,305.0	$1,843.0

Note: Figures represent billions.
Sources: Health Care Financing Administration; authors' estimates

share of total health care expenditures will continue to decline, reaching 29.7 percent by 2005. Physicians' share will remain nearly constant at just over 20 percent. Drugs and supplies will account for 11.1 percent, up from 9.4 percent in 2000.

What Factors Will Drive the Expected Increase in Health Care Spending?

Over the years we have read and heard many "experts" point to certain factors as being the most important in driving health care revenues to providers and suppliers or costs to payers. "It's the new medical technology." "We have too many hospital beds and too many specialists." More recently the focus has shifted to the proliferation of high-priced new drugs and the fact that pharmaceutical companies are spending almost $2 billion a year marketing directly to consumers. Others think it is fraud and abuse. The aging of the population is often viewed as the number one culprit. "Unrealistic consumer expectations" are frequently cited

**Table 4.2. National Health Care Expenditures by
Spending Category and GDP, 1995, 2000, and 2005.**

Spending Category	1995	2000	2005
Hospital care	$347.2	$387.2	$534.7
Physician services	201.9	255.4	366.4
Dental	45.0	60.0	82.0
Other professional services	53.6	78.0	114.0
Home health	29.1	39.0	56.5
Drugs and other nondurables	88.9	122.3	199.5
Vision products	13.1	16.0	20.7
Nursing home care	75.5	97.0	130.0
Other personal care	25.1	40.0	73.5
Program administration and net cost of private health insurance	53.3	87.0	118.5
Government public health	30.4	47.0	64.5
Research and construction	30.6	36.0	43.5
Total	$993.7	$1,264.9	$1,803.8
Prescription drugs only	$61.1	$90.0	
GDP	$7,270	$9,300	$151.0[a]
Total health care expenditures ÷ GDP	13.7%	13.5%	$11,2801

Note: Figures represent billions.
[a] Many in health care believe this estimate is too low.
Sources: Health Care Financing Administration; authors' estimates.

by physicians. We used to hear much talk of defensive medicine—performing marginally valuable tests—and inappropriate and unnecessary care. Exhibit 4.2 lists twenty factors that have been identified by various experts as the most important in driving health care costs.

How can there be *twenty* factors that are each the most important? There cannot be. Who is right? No single factor is dominant, but several are important. The next few paragraphs focus on several of these factors and analyze the ways in which they will continue to drive year-to-year increases in health care expenditures.

Figure 4.1. Distribution of National Health Care Spending on Various Services, 2000 and 2005.

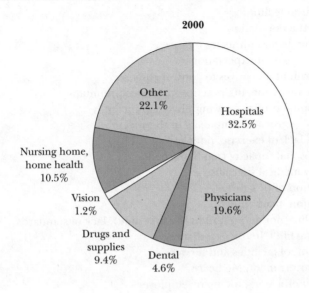

2000

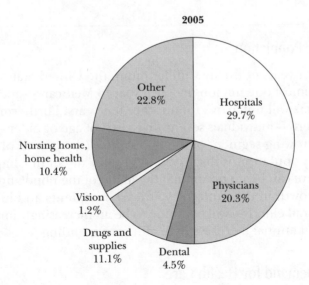

2005

Sources: Health Care Financing Administration; authors' estimates.

**Exhibit 4.2. The Twenty "Most Important" Factors
Driving Health Care Costs for Payers.**

1. New medical technology
2. Aging of the population
3. Inappropriate and unnecessary care
4. Unrealistic patient expectations
5. Lack of patient incentives to control costs
6. Defensive medicine, malpractice insurance premiums
7. High hospital profits, growing physician incomes
8. Insurance overhead, complexity of the system
9. Smoking, lack of exercise, poor eating habits
10. Excess hospital capacity (too many beds)
11. Too many medical specialists
12. Proliferation of new drugs
13. Competition, marketing
14. Poor quality (not doing it right the first time), lack of standards
15. Prolonging life ("heroic" medicine)
16. Duplication of facilities and services
17. Federal government, Medicare
18. Hospital inefficiency, too many employees
19. Mandated benefits
20. Fraud

Aging of the Population

In the earlier years of the new millennium, the United States will
be adding almost one million people a year to Medicare—and the
baby boomers will not arrive for another ten years! Furthermore,
the frail elderly—individuals seventy-five years of age or older—are
the fastest growing segment of the population (the growth of this
part of the population is discussed in greater detail in Chapter
Seven). There can be no doubt that the aging of the population—
equaling growth in the ranks of Medicare recipients and in the
number of frail elderly—will continue to be an increasingly important driver of annual increases in health care spending.

Insatiable Demand for Health Care

A hospital CEO we know often observes, "The demand for health
care in this country is insatiable." Although we have never argued

with him, we were not always sure we agreed. Why would anyone want to overuse the health care system? With each passing year, however, it seems more and more that his assessment of health care demand is correct. An increasing number of higher-income citizens are opting for cosmetic surgery and paying for it out of their pockets. Lifestyle drugs are selling at a record pace. As we discuss later in this chapter, consumers are the biggest growth sector of the health care marketplace.

Unrealistic Consumer Expectations

A favorite complaint of physicians is unrealistic consumer expectations, and they have a point. Most physicians can cite numerous examples of consumers demanding tests that were not medically warranted or requesting surgeries (for example, removal of a prostate when less invasive treatment options existed) that were of marginal value. Now, thanks largely to the onslaught of pharmaceutical advertising, a growing number of consumers are demanding name brand drugs instead of generics.

One of the themes of this book is that consumers are playing a growing role in health care decision making. Consumer expectations, already high in the United States, are going through the roof. However, we do not think this is necessarily bad, particularly when it comes to wanting better service, greater access, and more emphasis on prevention. Furthermore, if consumers are willing to pay for an increasing number of medical procedures and drugs not covered by insurance, they are likely to be more demanding of excellence in the delivery of services and in the results.

In short we believe that high consumer expectations are inevitable. This does not mean that physicians have to retreat in the face of demands for inappropriate and unnecessary care and prescribe name brand drugs when the generics would do just as well. At the same time, however, the consumer movement in health care is necessarily going to drive up health care spending.

Open-Ended Payment and Medicare

First-dollar coverage and the third-party payer system have historically insulated consumers from the cost of their health care.

Many physicians and managed care executives refer to the "entitlement" attitude of many consumers. Fee-for-service medicine, even the PPO variety with deep discounts for physicians and hospitals, offers only limited controls over utilization and thus drives year-to-year increases in health care spending. Despite predictions of growth, capitated payment represents a relatively small proportion of reimbursement for most physicians and medical groups, and it is unlikely to increase in importance (see Chapter Twelve).

Even though Medicare is viewed by some as a stingy payer, the truth is that this federal program has fueled much of the year-to-year growth in overall health care expenditures over the past decade. (This is discussed in detail in Chapter Five.)

The other side of this coin is reflected in the belief on the part of a number of HCFA economists that the "most important moderating influence for growth in health care costs is expected to be the slowdown projected for Medicare and Medicaid" (Smith and others, 1998, p. 137). One of the questions discussed in Chapter Eleven is whether or not Congress and the federal administration will be able to resist pressures to relax Medicare and Medicaid spending limits. We have serious questions about the ability of government to stand up under grassroots political pressure for improved payment, especially for hospitals.

Technology

One of the important points about the impact of technology on health care costs is that although there are few major technological breakthroughs that immediately affect spending, the application of technology spreads over time. Professor Victor Fuchs of Stanford notes, "The effect of technological advances on expenditures is rarely simple or immediate. Occasionally a blockbuster 'breakthrough' has a rapid impact on expenditures; Viagra, the new male impotence drug, for example, is expected to boost annual health care spending by more than a billion dollars within a year or two of introduction. More often, however, a technological advance such as a new drug, surgical procedure, or diagnostic technique has only a modest effect on expenditures initially. Over time, however, further development, refinement, and diffusion of the technology result in large increases in spending" (Fuchs, 1999, p. 13).

The use of advanced medical technology and massive investment in clinical information systems, likely to continue in the foreseeable future, will remain a major force pushing up health care spending. In fact, the evidence we consider in Chapters Eight and Nine suggests that advances in medical technology may be coming faster than at any time in the history of medicine. This is reflected in scenario 3 (presented in Chapter Thirteen).

The Medicare Payment Advisory Committee (MedPAC) "believes that hospitals should not be discouraged from adopting technologies that are necessary to maintain the high quality of care available to Medicare beneficiaries" (Medicare Payment Advisory Committee, 1999, p. 149). In our judgment consumers would not stand for anything less than an all-out effort to develop and apply medical technology.

Drugs

Here is what the *Wall Street Journal* said about the explosion in spending on drugs: "A revolution in pharmaceutical research, a billion-dollar marketing blitz and Americans' voracious appetite for Viagra, Claritin and a host of other pricey pills are driving drug spending to record-high levels. And nobody, it seems, knows what to do about it" (Tanouye, 1998, p. A1). The article goes on to say that for the Chrysler Corporation spending for employees' prescription drugs has risen 86 percent in five years. "At Blue Cross Blue Shield of Michigan, drug outlays now represent 28% of total expenditures—*more than the amount spent by the health plan on doctor visits.* . . . The pharmaceutical frenzy is expected to get worse in coming years, as drug giants crank out more new medications to salve an aging population. . . . On average, people over 65 fill between nine and a dozen prescriptions a year, compared with two or three for people between the ages of 25 and 44" (emphasis added).

The *Wall Street Journal* ran a series of articles on this subject, and the overall conclusion was that consumer demand for drugs is likely to drive one of the biggest health care spending sprees ever. We agree. (The matter of how to pay for these new drugs is discussed in Chapter Eleven.)

Complexity of the Health Care Industry

The pluralistic U.S. health care system carries a large—many would say excessive—bill for marketing, management, and administrative and financial services. Estimates of these costs range from 25 to 30 percent of all health care spending. This compares with less than 10 percent in Canada. By comparison Medicare has administrative costs of 2 percent (this does not include the added overhead for medical groups and hospitals).

Comparisons of Administrative Expenses

There have been a number of studies of the administrative expenses associated with the financing and delivery of health care in the United States. For example, in a 1993 study Steffie Woolhandler, David Himmelstein, and James Lewontin found that administrative costs accounted for 24.8 percent of the spending of 6,400 hospitals they studied. By comparison they found that hospital administrative expenses were more than twice those in Canada. Of course, this is one of the arguments often advanced by Woolhandler, Himmelstein, and others for a single-payer system like the Canadian one.

Impact of Health Care Administrative Complexity: An Example

Here is one very personal example of the inefficiencies in the administrative side of health care:

> Carolyn Boyer, a 50-year-old lawyer, has been battling breast cancer for nearly six years. And like so many patients, she's had another battle to wage on the side: with a never-ending barrage of insurance-payment foul-ups and medical billing mistakes. Time and again, her health plan, NYLCare Health Plans of the Mid-Atlantic, blundered with paperwork, misprocessing claims that resulted in initial denials of coverage for doctor visits and other services. Doctors and hospitals made their own mistakes, sending Ms. Boyer incomprehensible bills and over-due-payment notices for money

she didn't owe. Although the mistakes usually involved relatively small claims, they added up to thousands of dollars.

But her ordeal offers a stark look at the modern health-care bureaucracy, a snarl of so many players with so many conflicting rules that it's no wonder mistakes are so routine. For many patients with serious medical problems, the result is a nightmare that unfolds precisely when they are least able to cope with a new source of stress [Jeffrey, 1999, p. B1].

The article goes on to detail many instances of errors and buck passing among medical groups, hospitals, and health plans. This is an example of what we mean when we refer to the "complexity" of health care in the United States.

As long as we continue with a pluralistic system—large numbers of payers and numerous physician and hospital organizations— combined with a growing emphasis on consumers, the marketing and overhead expenses associated with health care will continue to climb. This anticipated growth in spending on the nonclinical side of health care is an argument for system simplification or a single-payer system.

Excess Supply of Physicians

The oversupply of physicians is a problem that has been getting worse (see Figure 4.2 for the trend in the number of physicians over the past twenty years). Despite numerous studies over the past two decades that have produced consistent results showing that the United States has too many physicians, mainly medical specialists, the flow has not slowed. Furthermore, the pipeline is full, with the number of applicants at medical schools showing no signs of abating.

Given this growing surplus, how are so many specialists able to survive economically? That is an interesting question. In our opinion Medicare keeps many specialists financially afloat by allowing recipients to use any physician—primary care or specialist—without restrictions. The movement of Medicare recipients into HMOs has the potential to change this dynamic, and we expect an increasing number of specialists who do not participate in Medicare risk contracting to get squeezed financially.

**Figure 4.2. Active Nonfederal Physicians
in the United States, 1980–2000.**

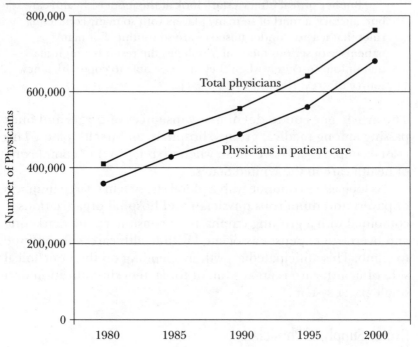

Source: Bureau of the Census figures and estimates.

There is little doubt that the excess supply of medical specialists and the ready availability of technology account for a significant
part of the reason why health care spending has been increasing
and will continue to grow rapidly in the future. Physician-induced
demand for health care services is a well-established pattern of behavior. The Wennberg studies discussed further on and the experience of many managed care organizations that have moved
medical specialists from fee-for-service payment to capitation provide ample evidence of this phenomenon.

We do not see the problem of a growing surplus of medical specialists easing anytime over the next five years. In fact, the problem
is likely to become more severe. Therefore the surplus of physicians
will continue to be an important factor driving year-to-year increases in health care spending.

Factors Likely to Be Less Important in the Future

There are four factors that may not be as important as they have been in the past in driving health care spending, which could result in a decline in health care industry revenues. They are (1) inappropriate and unnecessary care, (2) fraud and abuse, (3) surplus of hospital beds, and (4) "heroic" measures.

Inappropriate and Unnecessary Care

A growing emphasis on clinical guideline development and related efforts to establish a more rational basis for clinical decision making could slow clinical variation as a factor driving health care expenditures. Many large health care organizations and integrated systems have identified clinical guideline development as one of their core strategies for the future. These efforts are being supported by the development of clinical information systems. This combination could have a dampening effect on increases in health care revenues, especially in the period from 2003 to 2010.

Our optimism that the extent of unexplained regional variations in medical care may be coming down could also be wishful thinking. Recent reductions in clinical variation are not supported by the findings of Dr. John Wennberg and his colleagues at the Dartmouth Medical School (1996), as reported in *The Dartmouth Atlas of Health Care*. We can only hope that the future will be different.

Fraud and Abuse

This factor was highlighted in 1997 by the investigation of Columbia/HCA and has received a tremendous amount of attention over the past three years in the form of corporate compliance initiatives. The fact that some physicians and hospitals have been deliberately pushing the limits in billing Medicare and other payers has increased their health care revenues, at least through 1997.

Looking ahead, we do not anticipate health care spending getting much of a push from overly aggressive billing and collections approaches. Indeed, many hospitals and medical groups are going out of their way to be conservative. We know of one hospital that hesitated to implement a consultant's recommendation that they hire a firm to help with their billing. The CEO said, "We may be leaving a few hundred thousand dollars on the table each year, but none of us wants to risk getting into trouble with the Feds. Jail time is not appealing."

It also could be argued that the cost of corporate compliance will exceed the potential savings to payers. As the 1990s came to a close, many health care organizations were spending millions in their efforts to comply with increasingly complex federal and payer rules and regulations.

Surplus of Hospital Beds

The number of hospitals and staffed inpatient beds has been declining, although not fast enough to satisfy many critics. The United States has fewer hospital beds per hundred thousand residents than any of the Group of Seven (G7) countries (Canada, France, Germany, Italy, Japan, the United Kingdom, and the United States). Also, the percentage of the population admitted to a hospital each year in the United States is less than in any G7 country other than Japan, and average length of stay for those admitted for inpatient services is by far the lowest among the G7 countries (Anderson, 1997).

We do not expect hospital bed capacity to increase; therefore surplus beds are unlikely to be used to generate additional revenues for hospitals. In fact, with tight management by hospital boards and chief executives, the rational reduction in inpatient capacity should slow the rate of increase in health care spending. And, as noted in Chapter Three, spending on hospitals has declined as a percentage of all health care expenditures over the past twenty years.

"Heroic" Measures

We have heard claims from Richard Lamm, former governor of Colorado, and others that a significant portion of all health care dollars spent on a person are spent in the last twelve months of life. Of course, much of this effort is futile in terms of avoiding death although these expensive efforts may alleviate pain and suffering. On this point one physician told us, "You may be right, but how am I supposed to know which patients are going to get well and live longer and those that may pass on? You tell me how to figure that out, and we can save some money!"

There have been a number of studies suggesting that allegations of excessive spending to prolong life are overstated. For example, research by two physicians has concluded that the 2.17 million Americans who die annually contribute about 10 to 12 percent of all health care expenditures. The same research states, "The amount that might be saved by reducing the use of aggressive life-sustaining interventions for dying patients is at most 3.3 percent of total national health care expenditures" (Emanuel and Emanuel, 1994, pp. 542–543).

We believe that increased use of living wills mitigates against "heroic" measures to keep patients alive. Thanks to Governor Lamm and others, this issue has had extensive press coverage (as has his misunderstood statement that Americans have a "duty to die"). People are planning ahead, both for themselves and their loved ones. Therefore we do not view extensive measures to prolong life as a significant future driver of health care costs for Medicare and other payers.

The Most Important Factors Driving Health Care Spending in the Future

After weighing the evidence, we conclude that the most important factors driving spending in the health care industry over the next five years will be

1. *Increasing consumer expectations.* Spurred by widespread use of the Internet and drug company advertising, this is bound to be a major factor driving up health care spending. Although physicians often complain about unrealistic consumer expectations, consumer spending on health products and services is the bright spot of the future for many physicians and hospitals.
2. *New drugs.* This has to be near the top of any list of factors pushing up health care expenditures, and there is no slowdown in sight.
3. *Technology.* The availability and application of medical and information technology will become even more important than in the past. In some industries the application of technology leads to lower costs, but this is unlikely to happen in health care.

4. *Aging of the population.* The aging of Americans, including the longer life span of the frail elderly, continues to be an important driver of health care spending and one that is inevitable.

5. *Administrative expenses.* Given the growing complexity of the fragmented U.S. health care system, the overhead associated with health care financing and delivery is increasing.

6. *Surplus of physicians.* The problem is getting worse each year; therefore it will continue to drive up health care spending through physician-induced demand. Unfortunately, the result will almost certainly be a reduction in quality of care (for example, some specialists performing an insufficient number of procedures to maintain and improve their skill levels).

We believe that these six "drivers" will account for two-thirds of the projected annual increases in health care spending.

Conclusions

We expect annual increases in health care spending of 6 to 7 percent per year (about twice the expected growth rate of the CPI) over the first five years of the new millennium. This estimate is consistent with HCFA staff projections.

There are a number of pressures—technological advances, new drugs, consumer demand, aging of the population—that suggest health care spending will continue to grow from an estimated $1.3 trillion in 2000 to $1.8 trillion by 2005. Although there are some sources of downward pressure on health care budgets—Medicare spending limits coming from the BBA and more aggressive efforts to reduce clinical variation—we do not believe these will be sufficient to slow health care spending.

We are concerned about growing inequities in the U.S. health care system. We believe that the *unfairness* of the system is potentially more dangerous to the future of the present employer-based approach, dominated by managed care, than the fact that health care spending is moving toward 15 percent of GDP. This growing disparity between those who pay and those who receive health care benefits, which we believe is an important source of disequilibrium for health care, is the subject of Chapter Five.

Who Pays for Benefits and Who Receives Them

*The problem of cost shifting, more than anything else,
demonstrates the impending collision of market-based
strategies in the healthcare industry and policy-driven
concerns over the present state of the U.S. healthcare system.*

DEAN C. CODDINGTON, DAVID J. KEEN,
KEITH D. MOORE, AND RICHARD L. CLARKE,
The Crisis in Health Care, Jossey-Bass, 1990

Were we alarmists in 1990 in singling out cost shifting as a potential destabilizing factor in health care? What has happened over the past decade that has affected those who pay for health care services and those who receive the benefits? Where is health care cost shifting headed in the twenty-first century?

The wholesale move toward managed care provided employers with a defense against the huge costs that had been shifted to them in the 1980s during the heyday of indemnity insurance. Beginning about 1997, employers started shifting a larger portion of their health care costs to employees.

In the 1990s, however, growth in Medicare took much of the pressure off employers and individuals. In fact, during the period from 1990 to 1997, we would often hear medical specialists and hospital administrators in some parts of the country characterize Medicare as their best payer.

As we move into the new millennium, which groups are likely to be paying more than their fair share of the full costs of delivering health care services, and which segments are going to be subsidized? Has the large-scale cost shifting that threatened the viability of the health care system in the early 1990s been brought under control? If cost shifting threatens to get worse, will we find ways to limit this practice to more reasonable levels and achieve more equality between who pays and who benefits? Exhibit 5.1 highlights the major findings of this chapter.

Cost Shifting: Overview

Cost shifting—the shifting of a portion of direct and indirect expenses from one payer to another—is not limited to health care. Business travelers pay more for their airline tickets, and absorb a bigger share of airline overhead expenses, than do senior citizens and vacationers. In a supermarket certain products and brands are more profitable than others and carry a disproportionate share of the overhead. Corporations that purchase expensive skyboxes in new football stadiums subsidize ticket prices for fans sitting in the end zone.

Cost shifting in health care refers to the dollars different buyers, or groups of buyers, pay for the same mix and quantity of medical services. For example, we found in 1990 that employers paid $142 billion for health care services that had a full cost of

Exhibit 5.1. Highlights: Cost Shifting Leading to Destabilization.

- For much of the mid-1990s Medicare grew rapidly and took much of the cost-shifting pressure off employers.

- Just over 40 percent of the population—115 million Americans— receives 60 percent of the health care services and pays substantially less than full cost. This is likely to grow worse in the future, mainly because of the BBA and expected increases in the number of the uninsured.

- Managed care's ability to control employers' health care costs has been overrated. This raises questions about the ability of managed care to control employers' health benefit costs in the future.

- The inequities built into health care financing are likely to lead to more serious conflict than we have seen in the past and could lead to destabilization of the U.S. health care system.

$85 billion. Medicare, by contrast, paid $100 billion for medical services that cost $115 billion, including overhead (Coddington, Keen, Moore, and Clarke, 1990).

Cost Shifting in 1990 and 1995

We have often used the analogy of a balloon to illustrate cost shifting in health care. When you push on one part of a balloon, it either expands in another spot or it pops. Figure 5.1 shows how the health care cost-shifting balloon looked in 1990. Employers and employees were on the receiving end of most of the cost shifting handed out by hospitals and physicians, as providers tried hard to collect enough to cover their overhead and earn a reasonable return. Medicare, Medicaid, and the uninsured did not pay their fair share of full costs. Medicare's payments to hospitals led to negative margins from 1990 through 1992 (Medicare Payment Advisory Committee, 1999).

By 1995, however, with the growth of both managed care and Medicare, the bulges in the cost-shifting balloon had changed substantially, as Figure 5.1 shows. Medicare joined employers and consumers in subsidizing Medicaid recipients and the uninsured.

In 1995, hospital margins for Medicare patients were 10.8 percent (Medicare Payment Advisory Committee, 1999). On the outpatient side Medicare's payments to ambulatory surgery centers increased by 12 percent annually in the mid-1990s. During the same time, payments to hospital outpatient departments increased by 8 to 11 percent annually. All of this illustrates the financial impacts of Medicare, which became one of the best payers in the mid-1990s.

Mainly because Medicare began to pay its fair share, the amounts of physicians' and hospitals' overhead dollars that needed to be absorbed were less. Therefore physicians and hospitals had much less need to shift costs in the mid-1990s, and the financial performance of most providers was strong. In discussing cost shifting to Medicare, one physician told us, "I would agree that Medicare has been our best payer. However, I don't believe that physicians consciously shift costs to Medicare. It just turns out that since Medicare pays well right now, they bear most of the burden."

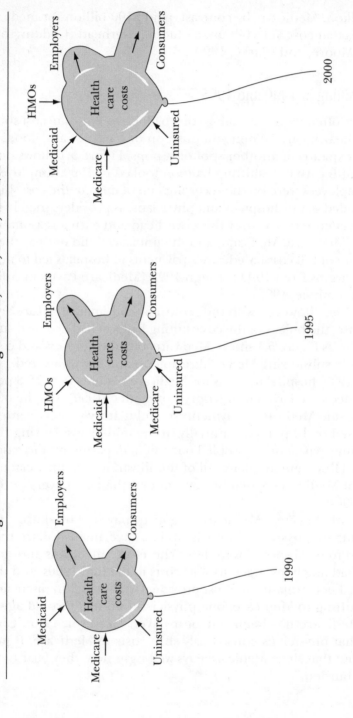

Figure 5.1. The Cost-Shifting Balloon, 1990, 1995, and 2000.

Cost Shifting in 2000

How has cost shifting, and the shape of the balloon, changed since 1997?

- The number of uninsured Americans continued to increase, reaching an estimated forty-five million in 2000.
- The BBA has, at least for the time being, slowed down Medicare's ability to maintain its position as an equitable payer of hospitals and physicians. This leaves the forty million (and growing) seniors and disabled paying a decreasing share of the full physician and hospital costs of providing medical services for them.
- The thirty million Medicaid recipients (excluding those in nursing homes) continue to pay 40 to 60 percent of the cost of the medical care they receive. Again, given the budget limitations of both federal and state governments, Medicaid is unlikely to pay a higher share of what it costs to meet the health care needs of this group.

This adds up to 115 million Americans—40.5 percent of the total population—who are either paying less than the full cost of health care services or moving in that direction (for example, Medicare under the BBA). Moreover, these 115 million receive an estimated 60 percent of the services of physicians, hospitals, and other providers. As the BBA fully kicks in over the next few years, the disparity between payments made for health care services for the Medicare population and the full cost of providing these services will grow larger.

As the decade of the 1990s drew to a close, there was little indemnity insurance left to pick up the slack. Other than Champus, this left employers, employees, self-insured individuals, and those who use their discretionary income to purchase discretionary medical services (like cosmetic surgery) to absorb much of the direct costs and overhead of medical groups and hospitals.

Working on behalf of employers, managed care plans have inherited the burden of keeping cost shifting at bay. Their response has not been encouraging: premiums up by 10 percent in 1999 and by even more in 2000. Consumers of course are having to pick up an increasing share of the costs unpaid by Medicare, Medicaid, and the uninsured, as depicted in Figure 5.1.

Cost Shifting in the Future

Just when consumers began to step forward—both voluntarily (for example, by buying new lifestyle drugs and a host of new medical products and procedures) and involuntarily (through increased copayments, deductibles, and share of monthly premiums)—price hikes for health care services began to accelerate. In other words the trend toward consumer-driven health care is likely to clash with the need for providers to shift an increasing share of their costs to employers (despite the resistance of managed care), employees, and individuals (such as through premiums paid by the self-insured or the portion of health care paid privately by Medicare recipients).

Will Managed Care Hold the Line?

As we look beyond managed care, a key question is whether HMOs and PPOs will be able to avoid large premium increases. Will managed care be effective in resisting cost-shifting pressures resulting from a slowdown in the growth of Medicare and Medicaid and the continuing pressures brought by the large pool of uninsured Americans? To shed light on this question, we will re-examine the experience of managed care in the 1990s.

Decline in Health Plan Premiums: Who Should Get the Credit?

Here is a typical comment about the impact of managed care: "Now that corporate health care costs have been abated by the increased competition brought on by managed care, employers have redirected much of the energy and resources they dedicated to health benefits management to attention to the quality of health care services" (HCIA, 1998, p. xiii). Although managed care takes much of the credit for holding down employers' health care costs in the period from 1990 to 1998, Medicare was an important contributor. How could that be? What's the connection?

Booming Medicare Market

As we noted previously, with Medicare paying its fair share of health care expenditures and generating an increasing volume of patient visits and medical procedures, there has been less pressure on physicians and hospitals to shift part of their overhead expenses to employers. In the 1990s Medicare allowed physicians and hospitals to generate the revenues they needed to cover their expenses without shifting a disproportionate amount of overhead to employers and individuals.

The total dollar growth of Medicare as a payment source for physicians and hospitals is shown in Figure 5.2. This growth reflects a combination of higher unit prices for services and increased volume. This was illustrated by our earlier comments about hospital profit margins from Medicare and the rapid increase in Medicare payments for both hospital outpatient services and ambulatory surgery centers. From a physician and hospital perspective Medicare has been a high-growth market for most of the past decade.

Figure 5.2. Medicare Outlays, Part A and Part B, 1980–2000.

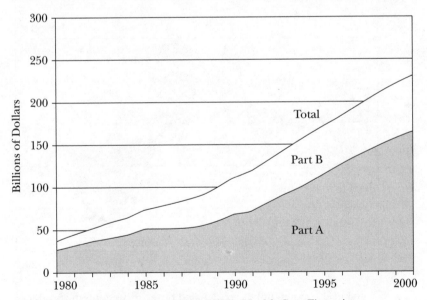

Sources: Office of the President (1980–1995); Health Care Financing Administration projections (1996–2000).

The growth of public funding (mainly Medicare) compared with the percentage rates of change for private sector employers for the period from 1980 to 2000 is shown in Figure 5.3. The darker shaded area in this figure shows that from 1989 through 1998, the rate of increase in public health care spending substantially exceeded that of private employers.

Figure 5.4 shows public and private rates of increase in health care spending combined with the overall rate of increase. The shaded area in Figure 5.4 reflects the ten years when rates of increase in public funding exceeded both the overall growth of health care spending and the health care spending of the private sector. Again, this supports the earlier point that Medicare has been a growth market—both in revenues and profitability—over the past decade.

Figure 5.3. Growth in Real Per Capita Private and Public National Health Expenditures, 1980–2000.

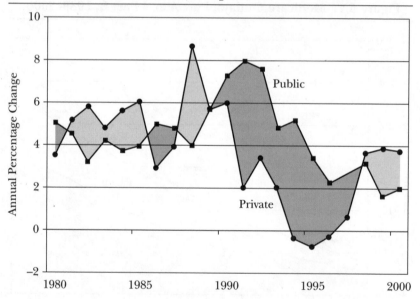

Note: National health expenditures are deflated by the gross domestic product deflator. The annual rates of change shown are real percentage changes, adjusted to reflect inflation.
Source: Smith and others, 1998, p. 131.

Does Medicare Seem a Growth Market Because Private Sector Spending Is Down?

Neil McLaughlin (1999, p. 58), managing editor of *Modern Health-care,* notes that managed care and Milliman & Robertson have done the dirty work of allocating health care resources: "They squeezed hospitals with such gusto that Medicare is now one of the best payers around." In our view Medicare was a growth market in the 1990s no matter what comparisons are used. Inflation-adjusted annual rates of increase have been in the range of 2 to 8 percent every year for the past two decades. The highest rates of increase were during the period from 1989 to 1994. John Iglehart (1999c, p. 302) agrees that Medicare was a growth market in the mid-1990s: "As private payments fell in relative terms, Medicare's payments rose faster than the costs of treating its beneficiaries. This phenomenon occurred over the period from 1994 through 1997, when Medicare was left untouched by budget cuts because

Figure 5.4. Annual Growth in Real Per Capita Private and Public National Health Expenditures, 1980–2000.

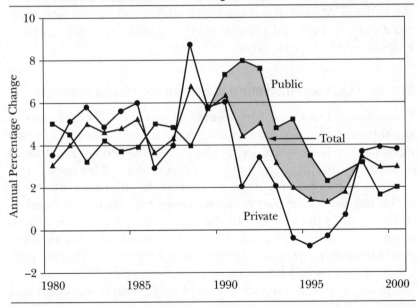

Note: National health expenditures are deflated by the gross domestic product deflator.
Source: Smith and others, 1998, p. 131.

Congress and the executive branch could not agree on new ways to slow its growth."

Government Viewpoint

Donna Shalala, secretary of health and human services, accused hospitals of using their generous Medicare inpatient profits to off-set the money-losing deals they arranged with HMOs. "Providers gave steep discounts to the private sector, assuming we'd never get our act together—but we did," Shalala said. "When we did that, they had no place to go for additional resources" (Hallam, 1999, p. 25). Shalala was referring to the government getting its act together by implementing the BBA.

Managed Care Receives Too Much Credit for Holding Down Employers' Health Care Costs

The fact that Medicare became a significantly better payment source for physician and hospital services in the mid-1990s was a contributing factor in lowering the rate of increase in employers' health plan premiums and costs. When managed care squeezed the balloon, Medicare was the bulge—a big one. Therefore managed care should not receive all the credit for holding down employers' health care costs.

Managed Care and the Future of Employers' Health Care Costs

Can managed care help employers to control health care costs in the future? Given the questions we have about the ability of managed care to limit costs, we doubt that managed care will be as effective in the future as many employers hope. Managed care's contribution to holding down employers' health care costs in the 1990s has been overstated. As managed care firms will need to improve their profitability in the early years of the new millennium, employers will probably not get much of a break. This could lead employers to engage in more direct contracting with medical groups and hospitals.

In markets with a significant surplus of medical specialists and a large population base, managed care may experience continuing success in limiting the rate of increase in hospital and physician spending. However, without expanded use of global capitation (fixed PMPM payment for all physicians), we do not foresee such success, at least not during the first few years of the new century.

Capitation is not the answer. Except in a few markets, capitation is not growing as a way of paying physicians or hospitals, and we do not believe this payment system will gain momentum.

Most of the recent growth in managed care enrollment has been in PPOs and open-access HMOs. In most markets the ability of these kinds of plans to hold down utilization and costs is suspect. The investment in infrastructure by these kinds of organizations, including sophisticated clinical and management information systems, has been limited.

Whereas all this may be good news for physicians and hospitals, it is terrible news for employers and consumers. If we are correct, *managed care must change significantly if it is to accomplish its objectives of containing costs and improving quality.*

How Will Consumers Fare?

If, as we predict, managed care experiences difficulty protecting employers from health care cost increases and Medicare and Medicaid are less attractive as payment sources, then consumers are in for a difficult time in the years ahead. The growing number of uninsured Americans exacerbates the situation.

As the decade of the 1990s closed, physicians and hospitals were just beginning to turn to consumers, seeing them as a source of funds to cover unabsorbed overhead expenses. Most of the highly publicized conflicts were between providers (physicians and hospitals) on the one hand and HCFA and managed care on the other. Hospitals were screaming—and lobbying heavily—for relief from the severe spending limits imposed by the BBA. With high fixed costs and a heavy dependence on Medicare, hospitals have been hit hardest by the BBA. There has been unprecedented conflict between physicians and managed care plans over control of patients (for example, disagreement over the role of primary care physicians) and payment arrangements.

Without relief at the national level—reasonable payment by Medicare and Medicaid and a payment source for the uninsured—the cost-shifting battle will be fought between managed care plans and employers and between employers and employees. Because we do not expect managed care to prevail in holding down employers' costs, *we believe there will be increasing pressure for employers to continue the long-term trend of shifting costs to employees.* One approach to doing this is through "defined contributions" (discussed in detail in Chapter Twelve).

If we are right in this prediction, the next five years promise to be challenging for physicians and hospitals but also to be a period of great opportunity for those organizations that make the right moves. The pressure on physicians and hospitals to satisfy consumers through better service, higher quality, and lower costs will accelerate.

Inequities in the Health Care System

Whenever a business announces its intention to downsize or the federal government talks about program reductions, most Americans say they can accept these changes if they are fair. Unfortunately, the U.S. health care system is anything but fair in terms of who pays and who benefits. The inequities between those who pay for health care and those who use health care resources are striking. As noted earlier, 40 percent of the population consumes two-thirds of the health care resources. What can be done to make the system more equitable and sustainable?

Universal Coverage

An important step would be to move toward universal coverage (a payment source for the uninsured, not a single-payer system). Uwe Reinhardt refers to the present approach to health care for the uninsured as "an informal, albeit unreliable, catastrophic health insurance program operated by hospitals and many physicians . . . who extract the premium for that insurance through higher charges to paying patients" (Iglehart, 1999a, p. 70).

Even if the payment levels provided for those in the uninsured pool were below those of Medicare and employers, universal coverage would represent a major step toward creating equity. When the combined federal-state CHIPS program is fully implemented, it will help alleviate the need for physicians and hospitals to shift their direct expenses and uncovered overhead to other payers.

Medicare Should Pay Its Fair Share

A second step would be to make sure that HCFA pays its fair share of the full costs of the health care services it purchases for Medicare recipients. This of course relates to the BBA and changes in the harshness of the financial reductions included in the original legislation.

As the largest single purchaser of health care services, Medicare has an obligation to pay amounts that approximate its share of full costs; if it does not, it runs the risk of seriously destabilizing the system. Agreeing with this, the MedPAC report said, "Medicare's payment systems should strive to establish payment rates that approximate the competitive prices that would prevail in the long run in local health care markets" (Medicare Payment Advisory Committee, 1999, p. 5). The reimbursement limits of the BBA are particularly devastating for rural hospitals, which typically have half or more of their patients on Medicare. These hospitals literally have no place to shift shortfalls in Medicare funding.

Since the mid-1980s health care has evolved into a heavily discounted business. Every payer wants a deal, and most seem to get it, at least on the surface. The fact is that no one even talks about "billed charges"; they are irrelevant. In any industry the largest customers cannot extract heavy discounts from suppliers without passing a burden on to smaller customers. If the smaller customers cannot afford to pay more, suppliers either go broke or get relief from their major customers. In health care this means that Medicare cannot expect employers and employees to pay disproportionately more while it pays less. (Medicaid and the uninsured are even poorer payers than Medicare, and this greatly aggravates the situation.) Those who will be hurt the most are physicians and hospitals who depend on Medicare as their largest customer and have nowhere else to shift costs.

Conclusions

The key conclusions of this chapter include the following:

- *Cost-shifting relationships change dynamically.* The nature of cost shifting from physicians and hospitals to different payer groups is not static; it changed dramatically between 1990 and 1995, and again between 1995 and 2000.

- *Medicare exercises enormous influence on the distribution of health care spending.* Medicare has been a source of substantial growth over the past decade, and many physicians and hospitals have been able to mitigate the cost pressures of managed care by shifting part of their uncovered overhead expenses to this federal program.

- *Managed care cannot be relied on to control costs.* Managed care's ability to hold down premiums for employers in the 1990s has been overstated. In our view, except in a few metropolitan areas, managed care has yet to prove that it can effectively contain costs. In fact, there is increasing evidence that managed care, with its high overhead and difficulties in controlling medical loss ratios, will be unable to significantly slow the rate of increase in employers' costs during the first five years of the new century.

- *Without appropriate federal action, inequities in health care financing will destabilize the system.* Looking ahead, if Congress and the federal administration stand behind the BBA, if Medicaid reimbursement rates are not improved, and if the number of uninsured Americans continues to increase, the inequities built into health care financing are likely to lead to more serious conflicts than we have seen in the past and a destabilization of the health care system.

Like it or not, consumers will have front-row seats to witness the battle over who pays for health care and who receives the benefits. If the movement toward consumer empowerment could be combined with fair payment by Medicare and at least partial payment on behalf of the uninsured, we could look forward to a period of stability and predictability in health care costs and improved quality and service.

The seven chapters in Part Three broaden this discussion by including a number of other factors likely to affect health care in the future: consumer empowerment; shifting demographics; information technology; genetic research and new drugs; consolidation of health plans, hospitals, and medical groups; and legislative and payment system changes.

External Factors Influencing the Health Care Marketplace of the Future

The healthcare industry faces a time of "fundamental economic discontinuity" that began in the mid-1990s, and managed care may be just the "most superficial" precursor of the kind of changes ahead. Medicare payment woes, escalating healthcare inflation, "unfunded liabilities" imposed by state and federal regulators, skyrocketing pharmaceutical costs, pressure from purchasers and consumers, and incursions by the Internet and other new technologies will make for tough times ahead.

DAVID LAWRENCE, CEO, KAISER PERMANENTE, quoted in *Modern Healthcare*, January 1999

Part Three covers what we consider to be the major external factors likely to affect health care over the first few years of the new century. Figure P.1 shows the factors considered in Part Three.

Part One set the stage for understanding the fundamental drivers of health care and managed care and the implications of these

Figure P.1. External Factors Affecting Health Care.

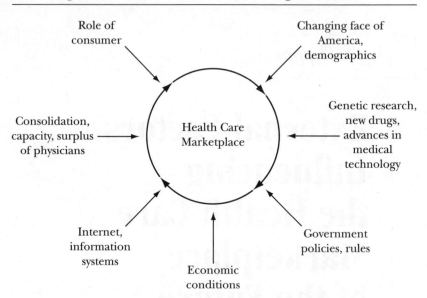

forces for the future. Part Two assessed the health care market-place with an emphasis on the size, shape, and future of the market. The seven chapters in Part Three continue our focus on important factors likely to shape the health care system of the future and set the stage for the development of the four scenarios presented in Part Four.

In Chapter Six we delve into a topic of great interest to all in health care—the increasing role of consumers in purchasing health care products and services out of their own pockets. The large pharmaceutical companies are certainly aware of this trend, and the rapid growth in pharmaceutical advertising aimed at consumers provides ample evidence of this shift in emphasis. The growth of cosmetic surgery, complementary and alternative medicine, and other medical services not covered by health plans or Medicare is truly impressive. We will consider how big this market is, how fast it is growing, and where it is headed.

Chapter Seven describes the changing demographics of the United States and the potential influence of these shifts on the demand for health care services in the future. We discuss the aging of the population, one of the most obvious and critical factors influencing the services the health care system has to deliver in the future. We also consider income, wealth, educational level, and the ability to pay for health care services.

We hear much about health care consumers being better educated and more interested in what health care products and services they are purchasing and consuming. For example, how big a factor will the Internet become as an aid to using the health care system? This is discussed in Chapter Eight. Other factors discussed in Chapter Eight include telemedicine and IT. We have believed for some time that the huge investments being made in IT would someday pay large dividends for patients and for those health care systems that successfully develop and implement clinical information systems with the ability to store, retrieve, and analyze medical information. Why is it taking so long to realize this dream? We know that some organizations now have clinical information systems in place. But what have been the results? What can we expect in the future? These questions are addressed in Chapter Eight.

Advances in medical technology and genetic research, leading to new drugs and therapies, hold great promise for mitigating the effects of many diseases and for nipping many others in the bud. What do these changes mean for managed care, for consumers, and for the health care system overall? What can patients expect? These issues are part of the discussion in Chapter Nine.

Chapter Ten focuses on the future implications of the consolidation of physicians, hospitals, and health plans. There is no doubt that health plans have been consolidating at a furious pace; we will consider the ramifications of this trend for physicians, medical groups, and hospitals. The surplus of medical specialists is an important and difficult factor to consider in terms of its impact on the future of health care. We put forth some thoughts on how this may play out.

Chapter Eleven deals with a number of important unresolved public policy issues, such as the uninsured, future funding of Medicare, and drug coverage.

Chapter Twelve identifies several potential payment models for the future. We discuss a number of possibilities, including increased use of defined contribution plans by employers, the Buyer's Health Care Action Group in the Twin Cities, MSAs, and individual-insurance models.

Chapter Six

The Growing Role of Consumers

The first wave of consumer-driven health care has been building slowly. As it accelerates in the next three years, it is necessary to understand where it is likely to rise first and what its impacts will be.

INSTITUTE FOR THE FUTURE, "Executive Summary: 'New' Health Care Consumer," May 1998

One of the basic themes of this book is that consumers are playing an increasingly important role in health care financing and decision making. We expect consumers to move into a position of dominance in health care during the early years of the new century. When it comes to the growing role of consumers in health care, we are often asked these questions:

- What makes you so sure that consumers are playing a larger role in health care and that their role will increase in the future?
- What is the evidence that consumers are willing to pay for additional choices and new products and services?
- Will consumers be willing to pay for the high-priced but improved drugs and the more advanced medical technology of the future, either indirectly through their health care coverage or directly out of their pockets?
- Will consumers have the right information when they need it and in a form they can understand?

The evidence of continuing growth in consumerism in health care is multifaceted. We have examined a variety of indicators, a few quantitative but mostly qualitative. One of the objectives of this chapter is to summarize the various factors we believe combine to point in the direction of a more consumer-driven health care system.

On the question about consumers' willingness to pay extra for certain health care services, we note the growth of many medical services not normally covered by Medicare or private health plans. The growth of complementary and alternative medicine (CAM) is further evidence of consumers' willingness to pay out of their pockets for products and services they desire.

The issue of whether consumers will be willing to pay for the new drugs and advanced medical technology of the future is more difficult to address. We believe that financing of new drugs and medical technology opens up opportunities for different types of health plans—more like catastrophic coverage, nursing home insurance, or Medigap insurance for seniors—that would cover these new products and procedures. The ability to pay for medical products and services is a function of income and net worth; the consumer market has to be segmented (which is done in Chapter Seven) to fully address this issue.

The question of whether consumers will have the information they need is a critical one to their health care purchasing decisions. We believe that they will have vastly more information in the future and that this information will be used in consumer decision making.

Of course, consumerism is not unique to health care. In fact, the growing role of consumers has been evident in other industries for many years. For example, the mutual fund industry developed largely in response to consumers' desires to invest in corporate debt or equities. The blurring of the lines between various types of financial institutions (such as commercial banks, savings and loan companies, and investment banks) and the success of home shopping networks on television are two other examples. Direct consumer purchasing of goods and services on the Internet, through Amazon.com for example, is just the latest example of consumers demanding more convenience, better service, and lower costs.

Consumerism in Health Care: Numerous Indicators

When health care first moved into the competitive and market-driven mode in the mid-1980s, we were often surprised to hear hospitals promoting their outpatient surgery centers or heart services on radio and TV. We knew that physicians controlled patients' selections of ambulatory surgery or cardiac services, such as cath labs. Our thinking at the time was that this type of health care advertising was institutional—designed to build awareness of the overall image of a hospital and its medical staff.

More recent health care advertising, whether it be for new drugs, ultrafast heart imaging centers, or vision correction surgery, is not institutional; it is intended to elicit a response from consumers. Given the huge amounts being spent on health-related advertising directly to consumers—we estimate it to be in excess of $3 billion per year—and the significant increase in consumer-driven decision making related to drugs and CAM, it must be working.

Our top indicators of the growing role of consumers in health care are summarized in Exhibit 6.1. This chapter summarizes each of these indicators of the growing influence of consumers in health care.

Direct-to-Consumer Marketing of Health Care Products and Services

Health care has flirted with direct-to-consumer marketing and advertising for years. Back in the early 1980s hospitals formed seniors' membership clubs to market services and build loyalty to the hospital system. The creation of heart, cancer, and women's health centers was an attempt by some health care systems to market directly to consumers by capitalizing on the favorable image of these kinds of high-profile clinical services. For obstetrics beautifully decorated birthing centers, candlelight dinners, and other amenities were promoted to expectant parents. Although these marketing efforts had some influence in attracting patients, the impact was limited because patients typically used the hospital their doctor recommended or where the doctor had staff privileges. More recently a physician's or hospital's affiliation with a health plan has been the key factor.

Exhibit 6.1. Indicators of Growth in Consumerism in Health Care.

1. Increased health care marketing and advertising directed at consumers.

2. The experience of many physicians and other health care professionals.

3. Backlash related to managed care restrictions (for example, gate-keepers and other cost management tactics of health plans) leading consumers to select health plans that offer more choice and fewer restrictions.

4. Greater use of cafeteria plans by employers. Related to this, there is increasing evidence that employers are considering defined contributions rather than defined benefits in their health plan coverage.

5. Surveys indicating that consumers are more satisfied with their health plans and providers when they have a choice of plans.

6. Rapid growth in spending on complementary and alternative medicines.

7. Changing demographics related to cultural, racial, and other shifts, such as the growing number of women with children, women who have had children, and seniors. These are the most knowledgeable and demanding health care consumers.

8. Growth in discretionary spending on health care services, such as laser vision correction surgery.

9. Increased consumer access to the Internet and high usage of health-related Web sites.

10. Resurgence of interest in self-care.

For many physicians and hospitals reorganization sidetracked customer focus. In the late 1980s and early 1990s many physicians and hospitals turned their attention inward, forming new partnerships, such as physician-hospital organizations, for single-signature contracting or to exert leverage on managed care plans. Customer focus got lost in the process of reorganizing and negotiating with large health plans.

Pharmaceutical Companies Set the Pace in Direct-to-Consumer Marketing

The pharmaceutical industry was among the first to recognize and capitalize on consumers' frustrations with the limitations of managed care plans and those plans' emphasis on drug formularies and generic drugs. Drug companies have traditionally marketed their products directly to physicians through "detail" representatives who call on physicians' offices, explain the latest drugs, leave plenty of samples, and often provide a free lunch for the doctors. By 1998 pharmaceutical companies were spending more dollars marketing directly to consumers than to providers, and this trend has continued into the new millennium. Changes in laws regulating advertising of pharmaceuticals paved the way for this to happen.

These direct marketing efforts continue to be successful for pharmaceutical companies. Spending on prescription drugs rose 85 percent over five years, reaching $102.5 billion in sales in retail pharmacies (Tanouye, 1998, p. A1). At the same time sales of generic drugs were flat. Conservative estimates of annual growth rates for drug sales during the initial five years of the twenty-first century are 15 to 17 percent per year.

Health Care Direct Marketing Efforts: Summary

Although not as hard hitting and pervasive as drug company advertising, other types of health care suppliers, health plans, hospitals, and medical groups are increasingly advertising and marketing directly to consumers. It is working; consumers are selecting physicians, health plans, and a wide variety of products and services that they learn about through advertising.

Feedback from Physicians and Other Health Care Professionals

Since the mid-1980s we have conducted over one hundred focus group sessions and hundreds of one-on-one interviews with physicians, other clinical staff, and those working in the management and financial side of health care. One of the common themes: consumers are becoming more knowledgeable and demanding. In fact, physicians often blame the high cost of health care on the "unrealistic expectations" of consumers.

Physicians' Perspectives

Here is what one senior physician told us: "When I first started in practice, patients would pretty much accept what I told them without much argument. However, this has been changing steadily over the past ten years, and it has reached the point where I expect to be challenged. Many of these patients are women who either have children or are a little older. They know quite a bit about health care, but they aren't as educated and sophisticated as they think when it comes to medical matters. They tend to overestimate their knowledge." This physician went on to say that the change does not bother him and that there is much good coming out of it. "At the same time it is going to make the practice of medicine in the future more challenging than it was during my career."

A family practice doctor told us, "When a patient comes in with the symptoms of a sprained ankle, I can pretty much diagnose the problem without taking X rays. I have seen hundreds of these kinds of cases. However, an increasing number of patients, particularly those who are younger, demand that I have it X-rayed. If I don't do it, they probably won't come back."

We have heard similar comments from many physicians. It is not difficult to sell physicians on the idea that consumers are becoming more demanding in many aspects of their health care.

Administrative and Financial Side of Health Care

The eight CFOs of large multihospital systems who participated in one of the roundtables conducted as part of writing this book were well aware of the growth in consumerism. One CFO said, "You don't have to convince us that consumers are playing a bigger role in health care decision making. We see it every day in terms of their demanding better services, more convenience, and greater choice. When they are paying all or part of the tab, they are especially diligent. I don't see it going back to the old days. If anything, consumers are becoming more sophisticated and even more demanding."

Consumers Opt for More Choice

As discussed in Chapter Two, the more restrictive HMOs had stopped growing in the late 1990s; most of the recent growth in managed care was in PPOs and POS HMOs. Anecdotal information from around the United States indicates that the trend toward selecting PPOs did not change as the 1990s ended. At the same time the proportion of employees choosing PPOs or POS HMOs increased substantially, with the number of enrollees surpassing the number enrolled in traditional HMOs (see Chapter Two).

All of this is evidence that consumers are paying more attention to the type of health plan they enroll in and that they favor those plans that offer more choice of physicians and hospitals. In some cases open-access plans are more expensive, but there is increasing evidence that the added cost is not an insurmountable barrier.

Employers Shift Risk and Decision Making to Employees

There are similarities between what happened to pension and profit-sharing plans over the past quarter century and what was developing with health insurance coverage in the late 1990s. Beginning in the 1970s and early 1980s, employers switched from defined retirement benefits to paying a percentage of income to employee pension plans, allowing employees to direct their own investments. Employers are now mostly off the hook for ensuring a specific dollar amount in monthly retirement benefits.

This shift in philosophy has been due to highly publicized examples of corporate underfunding of defined benefits and, on the other side of the coin, the opportunity for some organizations (including health systems) to recapture overfunding. Other factors that pushed corporations to change their approach in funding retirement programs included changes in IRS rules, the need for predictability of costs, and the diminished influence of unions.

Growth of Cafeteria Plans

When it comes to health care, increased use of cafeteria-type benefits plans is a step toward creating defined-contribution medical plans. Cafeteria plans offer employees a fixed amount per month or year from which they can choose the mix of benefits they desire. When the dollar amount of employees' choices exceeds the amount their employer will contribute, employees can elect to pay extra out of their pockets for benefits they desire.

Are Employers Opting out of Providing Health Benefits?

Some employers would prefer to go even further and get out of providing health benefits altogether. Speaking at the Health 2000

Forum in Seattle, Steven Hill, senior vice president of human relations at Weyerhaeuser Corp., said that "most employers would rather not be in the business of providing healthcare." He suggested that one of the main obstacles to creating a sustainable health care system is that "the people who use healthcare are not paying for healthcare." Many companies are already heading for the exit, he warned. "Look at the data. It's happening" ("Uncovered Lives," 1999, p. 64).

Defined Contributions Rather Than Defined Benefits

Although controversial, defined-contribution approaches are being seriously considered in both the private and public sectors. We believe this is evidence of the growing role of consumers in health care decision making. Several of the CFOs of large systems who participated in the roundtable discussion referred to earlier in the chapter said that large employers in their area were considering other options in order to control the cost of their health benefits. The CFO of a system that serves an industrialized area in the Upper Midwest said, "Employers look at their health benefit just like they do any other cost. If health care costs get back on the track they were on in the late 1980s and early 1990s, I don't think there is any question but that they will move to stabilize their costs. This will inevitably lead to clashes with labor unions, but the employers really have no choice." (Chapter Twelve presents substantially more background on both defined contributions and premium support.)

Surveys Show That Consumers Value Choice

On the question of consumers' attitudes toward choice in their health plans, a national study of the relationship between health plan satisfaction and choice concludes, "A growing body of literature suggests that a lack of insurance choices could be a core problem driving the public's dissatisfaction with health care" (Gawande and others, 1998, p. 184). Specific to the survey results, which were the focus of a *Health Affairs* article, the study found that "only a minority of the working-age population effectively control what health plan they get" (p. 184). "Persons without choice," the study determined, "were markedly more dissatisfied with their health plan, especially when enrolled in managed care" (p. 184).

Our view on the growing concern about freedom of choice is that many of the early enrollees in managed care plans did not place a high value on personal relationships with physicians. Although most managed care plans vehemently deny that they specifically target younger and healthier employees (in other words, that they cherry pick), we believe that employees with these characteristics often opt for HMO coverage. The data we have seen are mixed on this point.

However, given that something like 85 percent of all employees of organizations providing health benefits are enrolled in managed care plans, complaints about losing choice and the growing popularity of open-access and POS plans clearly demonstrate that we were too quick to conclude that consumers value small monthly savings more than freedom to choose their own health plan and physician. (Many in health care disagree with our conclusion and remain convinced that cost to employers and employees drives the market.)

Explosion in Complementary and Alternative Medicine

Nowhere is the power of the consumer more pronounced than in CAM, which has emerged as a result of growing consumer demand. "In an unusual twist, the CAM trend is led not by providers, insurers or technological advances; it is led by consumers seeking alternative approaches such as acupuncture, herbal therapy and chiropractic, to name a few" (Hofgard and Zipin, 1999, p. 16).

Growth of Complementary and Alternative Medicine

In 1993 Harvard physician David Eisenberg shocked the health care world with his study on the prevalence of the use of alternative medicine by Americans. Will Fifer, a partner in Clayton, Fifer Associates and a frequent speaker at Estes Park Institute meetings, summarizes Eisenberg's more recent research this way: "November 11, 1998, the second shoe dropped. On that date, in the *New England Journal*, Eisenberg et al. reported survey results indicating that their previous 1993 survey was no fluke—Americans were flocking to the altar of alternative medicine. The dramatic rise in the use of non-traditional medicine was due primarily to an increase in the proportion of the population seeking alternative care, rather than increased visits per patient" (Fifer, 1999, p. 1). Fifer continues, "Extrapolating these numbers to the entire U.S. population, 629 million visits were paid to alternative therapy practitioners, more than to all primary care physicians. . . . Alternative care has not 'replaced' traditional, science-based care; it has merely created a giant new industry devoted to healing rather than curing" (p. 1).

Eisenberg estimated the size of CAM at $13.7 billion in 1990. It was estimated that CAM out-of-pocket spending in 1997 was double this amount, or at least $27 billion. Others estimate that CAM spending was in excess of $50 billion in 1999 (Hofgard and Zipin, 1999). Spending on CAM is not included in the $1.3 trillion health care budget for 2000.

Users of Complementary and Alternative Medicine

Surveys of users of alternative therapies find that the largest segment consists of women who are well educated, above average in income, and between the ages of twenty-five and forty-nine (Windhorst, 1998). As discussed in Chapter Seven, this is one of the fastest growing population segments in the United States.

Another study notes, "Although educated, middle-class white persons between the ages of 25 and 49 years were the most likely ones to use alternative medicine, use was not confined to any particular segment of the population" (Astin, 1998, p. 1548). This research also concludes that users of CAM often hold to a philosophical orientation toward health that can be described as holistic (that is, they believe in the importance of body, mind, and spirit in health).

Consumers Do Not Discuss Complementary and Alternative Medicine with Physicians

Most people do not discuss their use of CAM with their traditional physician. Many people are going directly to the Internet or other sources to learn about treatments. The Internet has been a powerful tool for marketing dietary supplements and other alternative medicines. Furthermore, because herbal supplements are largely unregulated, advertisers can easily make health claims that may or may not be true.

Traditional Medicine Begins to Take Complementary and Alternative Medicine Seriously

Consumer demand for CAM has been so significant that Western medicine is taking the trend seriously. Residency programs now include rotations in CAM, and over three-fourths of medical schools include instruction in CAM. Researchers and physicians across the country are increasingly involved in conducting clinical trials to test the validity of the claims of CAM. The National Institutes of Health budgeted more than $50 million in funding for research on the subject in fiscal year 1999, compared with $2 million in 1992 ("1999 Industry Outlook," 1999).

Consumers Drive Growth and Acceptance of Complementary and Alternative Medicine

Consumers are pressuring health plans and employers into offering CAM benefits. In some parts of the country managed care plans are responding by adding CAM benefits to their plan designs. In addition, a growing number of self-insured employers are offering coverage for alternative medicine therapies ("1999 Industry Outlook," 1999). The rapid growth, huge size, and acceptance of CAM are important indicators that consumers are taking health care into their own hands, even if it means seeing practitioners other than their traditional providers (and not telling them about it) and paying most of the cost out of their pockets.

Changing Demographics Favor Those Interested in and Able to Finance Their Health Care

When we conclude that consumers are playing an ever-increasing role in health care, we are not talking about everyone. The lack of early success in signing up children for the CHIPS program is one indication that a number of parents either do not care or are incapable of handling the administrative burdens of enrolling their children in this program. Men between the ages of eighteen and fifty are not known for their interest in health. In contrast, our research, supported by that of many others, continues to show that women with children are among the most motivated and sophisti-cated health care consumers. Older women are also interested in health care, and many men, once they reach sixty-five years of age, suddenly develop a keener interest in their health.

Chapter Seven segments the consumer market by age, income, education, and family status. Our analysis shows that the number of people in the age, family status, and income categories most interested in health care are also growing the most rapidly.

When we say that consumers are playing a bigger role in health care decision making and finance, we are talking about key seg-ments of the population with the income and net worth to have significant impact. This group accounts for over half of the U.S. population and is growing rapidly.

Private-Pay Health Services Add Up

The burgeoning private-pay market for elective procedures pro-vides some of the most compelling evidence of the force of con-sumers in health care. Pick up any copy of *Glamour* magazine or *Men's Health,* and you will see pages of advertisements encourag-ing readers to enlarge their breasts, retard balding, correct their vision, improve their smile, or relieve stress through herbs, mas-sage therapy, acupuncture—you name it.

Cosmetic Surgery

We first realized the immensity of this private-pay market when we were working with a group of plastic surgeons. In a few short years the mix of procedures among the five thousand board-certified plastic surgeons in this country has shifted from 60 percent recon-structive work (involving such things as congenital deformities, trauma, and breast reconstruction) and 40 percent cosmetic to just the reverse. Demand for cosmetic surgery has never been greater—so much so that other medical specialists are getting into the busi-ness in record numbers (much to the dismay of board-certified plastic surgeons).

Nearly all aesthetic surgery is paid for directly by consumers. Financing companies have even sprung up to help consumers at all income levels finance their $5,000 face-lift or $7,500 tummy tuck. The market for cosmetic surgery is largely middle-aged women but not just the wealthy—a large portion of middle-income women also find their way into the cosmetic surgeon's office.

Improving Vision

Among the most popular medical procedures (and growing in popularity) is vision correction through laser surgery. The radio airwaves are crammed with advertisements for various surgeons and vision centers, and the procedure is predominantly private pay. Many consumers are finding this $2,000 per eye procedure to be well worth the cost. Since the Food and Drug Administration approved the excimer laser in 1995, the volume of laser eye procedures has increased dramatically. There were 70,000 procedures in 1996, 200,000 in 1997, and 350,000 to 400,000 in 1998 (Maller, 1999). Many factors continue to contribute to this growth. "Perhaps most notable," one article observes, "is the increase in consumer awareness of refractive surgery as a viable vision correction option along with the public's acceptance of in situ keratomileusis (LASIK) as a preferred treatment modality. In addition, expanded treatment options (i.e., FDA approval of its use in the treatment of astigmatism and hyperopia) will help market growth. Improved access to excimer lasers (i.e., availability of transportable lasers and open-access laser centers) is also contributing to the surge in refractive procedure volume" (Maller, 1999, p. 49).

Hearing Aids

The predominantly private-pay hearing aid business has been growing and is preparing for significant future growth. "The baby boomers are at the age when hearing loss becomes important. In addition to higher-quality hearing aids, they want those that are more cosmetically attractive. The number of hearing aids sold, and unit prices, have been going up, and we expect this to continue" (conversation with Bruce Schachterle, Mar. 29, 1999).

In 1998 a survey of audiologists found that a record 60 percent of those fitted with hearing aids were first-time users. The survey also indicated that the market had been growing for the past four years, and even higher growth rates were anticipated for the future. The sophistication and high-tech features of the hearing aids sold have also increased. The majority of audiologists surveyed reported that over half of the hearing aids they dispense have automatic signal processing, and a high proportion have programmable features (Kirkwood, 1999). This trend is expected to continue. The price of hearing aids has also increased and continues to move up. Between 1997 and 1998 the average price of a single hearing aid increased from $971 to $1,143, up 17 percent (Kirkwood, 1999). A set of hearing aids can easily cost over $4,000, and practically none of this expense is covered by insurance.

Fertility Services

Fertility testing, in vitro fertilization, artificial insemination, and a host of other services for would-be parents represent a rapidly growing private-pay market (as one of the authors well knows, having contributed $5,000 toward the $15,000 cost of in vitro fertilization for his daughter-in-law).

In vitro fertilization is barely two decades old:

> On July 25, 1978, as hundreds of reporters descended on the sleepy English mill town of Oldham, the 65-year-old obstetrician (Dr. Patrick Steptoe) delivered the world's first "test-tube baby," a healthy 5-lb. 12-oz. girl aptly named Louise Joy Brown. Conceived in a lab dish, or in vitro, from the egg and sperm of a working-class couple who had tried for years to have a child, she seemed as miraculous as any baby in 2,000 years.
>
> Today such artificially assisted pregnancies are commonplace (an estimated 300,000 have taken place in the past 20 years) and are only one of many options available to would-be parents—from using frozen embryos and surrogate mothers to picking the number, sex, and genes of their babies [Golden, 1999b, p. 178].

Long-Term Care

Many frail elderly and their families are choosing assisted living over nursing homes. The vast majority of assisted living is private pay, compared with a relatively small proportion of nursing home care that comes from private resources (most nursing home care is paid by Medicaid). There are over thirty thousand units of assisted living in the United States, charging anywhere from $1,500 to $3,500 per month for housing and personal care services. This has significantly cut into the private sector funds available to nursing homes. The cost of homemaker services, adult day programs, and other services that help individuals maintain health and independence in their own residential setting is largely borne by consumers.

The Internet as a Source of Medical Information

The Internet is behind much of the increased consumer demand for information and consumers' growing tendency to actively use that information. In fact, the rate of adoption of Internet technology in the home has far outpaced that of one of the most venerable fixtures in every home—the television.

A study of on-line users found that 43 percent of Internet users had accessed medical information in the previous twelve months. The count of health-related Internet sites is out of date as soon as it is reported. One source (Brown, 1998) estimated there were one hundred thousand health-related Web sites. Health care information seekers are older and better educated than the average adult Internet user. The typical profile is someone who is thirty-eight years old and has a college degree, an income of $55,700 a year, and a white-collar job. Two in five are women. These Internet users are mostly looking for information for themselves but also search the Web for information related to spouses', parents', and children's health issues. Favorite topics to research include alternative medicine, nutrition, women's health, cancer, and heart disease.

Andrew Grove, the founder of Intel and a survivor of prostate cancer, agrees that the Internet is bringing revolutionary changes to health care. Grove (Intel Corp., 1998) noted that health care faces an Internet-driven "strategic inflection point," a time in which extreme change alters the competitive landscape in an industry, creating both opportunities and challenges.

Internet Support Groups

Speaking of his own experience in attempting to find information on prostate cancer when his was first diagnosed in 1994, Andrew Grove (Intel Corp., 1998) said, "I found basic information, reviewed papers written by some pretty prominent doctors, but more importantly, I rapidly stumbled on what in today's terminology would be described as a support group, where patients were exchanging information and describing their experience with different treatments and different medical procedures." Grove went on to describe how the information and the ability to exchange information were vitally important. He said that his experience helped him realize the power of the Internet as a source of medical information and support for people anywhere in the world.

America Online's America's Doctor

By the end of 1998, America Online's America's Doctor Web site contained 6,700 articles that consumers could download, print, and e-mail to a friend, frequently asked questions, a news service, a wire service that was updated every fifteen minutes, and a listing of special health care events. Scott Rifkin, founder and CEO of America's Doctor, said, "The area we're the most proud of that is unique is 'The Doctor Is In' area. The consumer has the ability to go into this area, select a topic—children's health, women's health, pharmaceutical questions, dietary—and speak to a physician, pharmacist or dietician" (Intel Corp., 1998). Rifkin reported that the average wait time has been five to ten minutes. "We actually have a large number of physicians who are online answering these questions very quickly," Rifkin said. He added, "We expected to get 1,000 consumers per day accessing this site. We've had an average of 4,800 consumers per day with little promotion ourselves."

Dealing with a Personal Health Crisis

David Gustafson, professor of engineering and medicine at the University of Wisconsin, heads the Comprehensive Health Enhancement Support System (CHESS), a computer system that uses the Internet to provide support and information for people with serious diseases or medical crises. According to Gustafson (Intel Corp., 1998):

> The idea behind CHESS really is to focus on people who are going through a health crisis. When a person is diagnosed with a life-threatening disease, they go into a crisis mode. They desperately need information, they desperately need to talk to other people like them who are going through the same problem that they're going through. . . .

We take computers into the homes of women who are diagnosed with breast cancer, or people who have been diagnosed with
heart disease, and so on, and we leave the computers there for
somewhere between three and eight months.

Gustafson says that the CHESS program delivers the computer,
installs it, and trains the individual. Here is the testimony of a
breast cancer patient who lives in South Chicago: "At the time I
was diagnosed with my cancer, someone called me on the telephone and told me about CHESS program, a computer program
that all I had to do was just set it on my table at my house and I
could actually talk to other people on it. And it's like having a doctor in your own home. . . . you can ask any question that you can
think of. And before you go to sleep that night, the majority of
your questions are going to be answered."

When asked how most people like this program, Gustafson
replied that "the subjective impact has really been powerful."
Gustafson also noted that older people and those with lower levels
of education perform just as well as people with higher education.
"They use it as much," he explained, "and their quality of life goes
up at least as much."

Self-Care on the Rise

A friend told us that self-care was important when he was working
on his master's degree in health administration in the early 1980s:
"This is what we were to prepare for—a loss of patients in the hospital because people were going to do more on their own." He
went on to point out that this was one of many anticipated changes
in health care that never happened. However, the adage that what
goes around comes around may be true for self-care. Many
decades ago self-care—everything from at-home childbirth to
grandma's favorite treatment for ailments—was the norm. A
recently retired hospital CEO told us, "I remember my mother's
'doctor book.' Whenever one of the kids had anything wrong, she
consulted this well-worn, loose-leaf book. We couldn't afford to go
to a doctor unless it was an extreme emergency. Her approach
worked pretty well."

As American society has become more specialized and as the pace and complication of life have increased, the country has moved away from self-care. The worried working mother needs answers about her child's illness immediately, so she carts him off to the pediatrician as soon as she can get an appointment. With the growth of managed care, there have been increasing efforts to manage demand for medical services by encouraging self-care. A whole new health care services field that did not exist ten years ago—demand management—has emerged.

Chronic Diseases Lend Themselves to Self-Care

The rapid growth in the number of people with chronic medical conditions also gives rise to an increased interest in self-care. Physicians and other health care providers increasingly realize that lifestyle, income, and type of occupation have at least as much impact on health status as age or genetics does. Many chronic conditions, such as high blood pressure, diabetes, and heart disease, can be controlled by exercise, proper diet, and avoiding alcohol, tobacco, and other harmful substances. The MacArthur Foundation produced a study on successful aging that concluded longevity and vitality are more heavily influenced by lifestyle than by genetics. The report found that "only 30 percent is genetic. The other 70 percent is attributable to disease avoidance, exercise of mind and body and staying involved in life" (Deets, 1999, p. 28).

Some health plans, like Kaiser Permanente and Group Health Cooperative of Puget Sound, have been promoting the concept of an informed consumer for decades. The idea of preventive care and health education were at the root of the early HMOs. As noted in Chapter Two, one of the founding principles of Kaiser Permanente was that prevention and early intervention paid off, both in terms of medical outcomes and in cost savings.

Self-Care Products Fill Market Niche

Healthwise is a nonprofit organization created in 1975 for the express purpose of empowering consumers with information. The following is an excerpt from the promotional material of Healthwise: "Consumer attitudes and expectations toward choice, control and information [are] driving the transformation of the American healthcare system. The future belongs to those healthcare organizations that can put informed and empowered consumers at the very center of healthcare decision-making" (Mettler, 1999b).

Among its various services, the organization produces the *Healthwise Handbook,* a self-care guide to over 180 medical conditions. The handbook is tailored to the needs of sponsoring organizations. For example, Kaiser Permanente distributes the guide to every member, complete with the Kaiser logo and information on when members should call their Kaiser Permanente advice nurse.

Healthwise was able to put the concept of an informed consumer into practice through a grant from the Robert Wood Johnson Foundation and a pilot program in four counties in Idaho. Everyone in the area received a free copy of the *Healthwise Handbook.* All county residents had access to a Web site that directed them to more information and resources. An extensive community awareness campaign was run during the course of the pilot program. The goal was to determine what impact informed consumers would have on health care costs and use of the health care system. The study sought to include not just the baby boomers who actively seek out health care information but everyone in the community—from the single mom dependent on welfare to the local gas station attendant (Mettler, 1999a).

Over a multiyear period the pilot program was able to involve 70 percent of the community as active participants in the health awareness program. Surveys indicated that 85 percent of physicians supported the effort. Most important, the program created behavioral changes and cost savings.

Consumerism in Health Care: Summary

Based on the evidence presented in this chapter, it is clear that consumers are playing a much bigger role in health care decision making and that this will be one of the major trends of the first five years of the new millennium. Exhibit 6.2, which lists five consumer imperatives suggested by the Institute for the Future, summarizes the growing role of consumers in health care.

An increased emphasis on informed and empowered consumers leads to an important question: Will there be a slowdown in the rate of increase in health care spending, or will spending go off the charts?

Exhibit 6.2. Five Consumer Imperatives.

1. *Choice.* New consumers want to be involved in all types of choices related to their health care, including choice of plans, providers, and treatments.

2. *Control.* New consumers are more active, more engaged, and more involved in their health care.

3. *Customer service.* New consumers will demand from their health care services the same superior customer service they demand from retail and finance.

4. *Branding.* Given the overwhelming glut of information new consumers face, strong brands will cut through to reach them.

5. *Information.* New consumers are hungry for current, accurate, and understandable information about their health and health care. When they do not get it, they become frustrated.

Source: Institute for the Future, 1998.

Signs That Health Care Spending Will Grow with Consumerism

We believe that, to date, increasing consumer involvement has driven up health care spending. As noted earlier, it is not unusual for patients to demand a certain treatment even if it goes against the doctor's better judgment or is more costly than another suitable treatment. Doctors are forced into the uncomfortable position of having to debate with their patients or give in to their demands to avoid losing their business. We also believe that consumer spending on health care products and services not covered by health plans has exploded and is likely to continue to grow as long as the economy stays strong, income levels are high, and there are no major discontinuities in the equity markets.

Arguments That Greater Consumer Involvement Will Decrease Health Care Spending

There is the old argument that if consumers were spending their own money on health care, the size of the industry would shrink dramatically. In the next few years we may have a chance to find out whether or not this is true. (Chapter Twelve summarizes the trend toward payment models that emphasize greater consumer financial responsibility.) In at least one area consumer empowerment shows signs of containing health care costs. Living wills and advance directives are specifically aimed at encouraging consumers to make decisions about end-of-life care themselves. Research indicates that advance directives reduce hospital costs for terminal patients from $49,900 to $31,200 (Weeks, Kofoed, Wallace, and Welch, 1994).

Will Educating Consumers on Treatment Options Save Money?

Giving consumers knowledge and a choice of treatment alternatives does not mean they will always select the most costly or high-tech option. In fact, in many instances just the opposite occurs. Kaiser Permanente pioneered the use of educational videotapes and counseling on the treatment options for prostate cancer. Presented with the research and probabilities associated with various treatment options, patients are able to make informed choices based on what they believe is best for themselves and family members.

Under these circumstances patients often choose a more conservative, less costly treatment option. For example, at Kaiser Permanente the rate of prostate surgery among members has declined. Member response to the program continues to be enthusiastic. Similar stories abound regarding treatment options for cancer patients, back pain, and other conditions for which a range of treatment options exist. Informed consumers often prefer the less invasive (and less costly) treatment approaches.

We acknowledge, however, that there are differences of opinion on this issue. Some would argue that consumers, with a limited knowledge base, may demand treatment options that are not the most appropriate.

Conclusions

The movement toward consumerism in health care is far-reaching and will permanently change how health care services are accessed, financed, and delivered. Consumer expectations will fuel demand for more and better services. Assuming a continued strong economy, consumers will be willing to pay for the health care services they want, or they will demand that third-party payers step up to the plate to share in the cost.

A recession or stock market crash could pose a serious threat to the consumer movement in health care. Elective care and private-pay resources would decline whereas self-care and less costly CAM would expand as individuals adjust to their new economic circumstances. (This is part of scenario 2, discussed in Chapter Thirteen.)

Given the complexity of the health care system and its continued fragmentation, physicians, hospitals, and other health care providers will need to differentiate themselves and better understand and target relevant categories of consumers (the providers' market segments). Chapter Seven assesses the size, growth, and health care needs of various market segments.

The Changing Face of America

The baby boomers have transformed every industry they've touched. And the boomers are now aging into life stages where their concerns about health and their utilization of health services will become an increasingly important aspect of their lives.

MARY HASSETT AND MICHAEL RYBARSKI,
"Transforming and Repositioning Healthcare for the Boomers," *Healthcare Strategist*, February 1999

This chapter presents a framework for evaluating the various consumer market segments and how they will affect the financing and delivery of health care in the new millennium. Here are the issues discussed:

- Consumer market segments most relevant to the future direction of health care
- Seniors, especially the frail elderly, and their health care needs
- Income and net worth as factors in consumer use of the health care system
- Cultural diversity and urban and rural differences in the health care market
- Those with chronic illnesses and their part in the health care market
- Impact of the baby boomers on the health care market

Exhibit 7.1 highlights some of the findings of this chapter.

Exhibit 7.1. Highlights: The Changing Face of America.

- The two largest health care market segments are married couples with children and singles under sixty-five years of age; these two groups account for over fifty million households, or more than half of all households.

- Married couples with children (one-quarter of all households) account for 38 percent of all personal income.

- Market segments that have health insurance or Medicare coverage and substantial purchasing power represent 70 percent of the population. This suggests a large and growing market for discretionary medical products and services.

- Substantial regional differences exist in the quantity of health care services consumed.

- One hundred million Americans suffer from chronic illnesses, one-quarter of these disabling.

Segmenting the Health Care Market

In a consumer-oriented environment, market segments are best defined by distinguishing characteristics that set one group apart from another with respect to purchasing decisions. For example, some consumers are very loyal to their physician—they will travel greater distances or endure long waits to see a particular provider. Others are more interested in convenience, and the choice of provider is less important than the hours of operation, location, or how soon they can see a physician.

From a broad perspective we know that the two most important factors that influence use of the health care system are age and income. For example, it is now an oft-quoted statistic that individuals sixty-five and over typically account for three to five times the annual health care expenditures of individuals under sixty-five. We also know that the consumption of health care services rises with income. Higher-income households typically spare no expense when it comes to obtaining the best care, new drugs, or the benefits of the latest medical technology.

Our discussion focuses on the factors that most influence how health care services are used. In addition to age and income several variables play significant roles in how someone accesses health care services: gender, presence or absence of children, education, and geographical location (see Figure 7.1).

Segmenting the Market by Age and Income

We first look at age and income in the context of household type. The household is a relevant unit for the purpose of market segmentation because health coverage is often available at the family level, and this is where most medical decisions are made. Figure 7.2 characterizes the consumer market by household type, age, and income as of 1996.

Married Couples with Children

The largest group in sheer numbers and the one that draws the most attention from policymakers and employers is the nuclear family—married couples with minor children. Yet even this segment constitutes just one in four households in the United States.

Figure 7.1. Key Factors That Define Market Segments in Health Care.

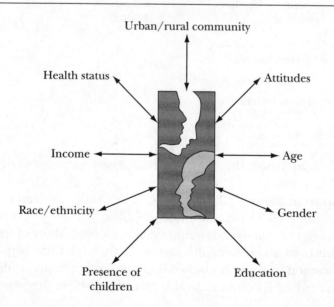

Figure 7.2. The Composition of American Households, 1996.

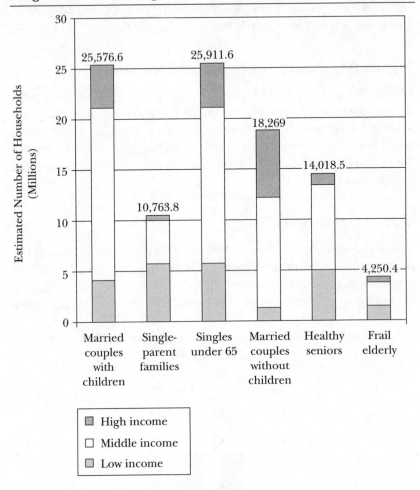

Source: McNeil, 1998, p. 9.

By way of comparison this segment comprised 41 percent of all households in 1969.

As shown in Figure 7.3, married couples with children command an estimated 38 percent of disposable income—disproportionately high compared with their overall numbers. Many of these households have access to health insurance through their employers. The women in these households are typically the major decision makers when it comes to health care. They select the plan (if

**Figure 7.3. Household Income by Various Types
of Households, 1996.**

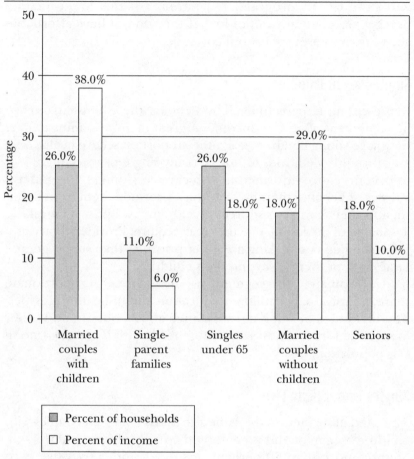

Source: McNeil, 1998, p. 9.

they have a choice), the doctors, and how their family will use the
system of care. They are in the driver's seat. Many of these households are also highly educated and well informed about the effects
of lifestyles on health. When we talk about consumers taking
charge of health care, this is a key group.

About 15 percent of this segment are the "spare no expense
for medical services" group, and they can afford to do so. A nearly
equal percentage of married couples with children are either

uninsured or underinsured. Their children might qualify for some form of publicly subsidized health benefit, like the new federal and state CHIPS program, but parents in this lower-income bracket are generally out of luck if they do not have affordable access to employer-sponsored coverage.

Single-Parent Families

Representing 11 percent of all households, these households earn just 6 percent of all U.S. income. A great many are uninsured. If they have young children, a significant portion secure health benefits through Medicaid. Although many single parents might like to become more informed health care consumers, the general stresses of keeping their lives on track preclude them from doing so, and their limited resources give them few options for taking advantage of the knowledge they may acquire. Provider choice and informed decision making are lower priorities than simply getting basic care for themselves and their children.

Unfortunately, this segment also includes a disproportionate share of individuals with lower education and unhealthy lifestyles. The incidence of smoking, substance abuse, obesity, and other lifestyle factors that adversely influence health is greater among this population.

Singles Under Sixty-Five

This market segment is the same size as the "married couples with children" segment and is composed equally of men and women. Slightly more than 60 percent of singles under sixty-five earn middle incomes. Most are working, have some access to employer-sponsored health care coverage, and are relatively young. Given the trends of marrying later in life and higher divorce rates, this group has grown over the decades. However, over a period of time they are likely to join the ranks of households with children.

The female households in this segment generally are health conscious, are particular about their health care, and have high expectations of service and quality. Although individuals in this market segment are likely not to have yet achieved their peak earning capacity, they earn a fair share of personal income and tend to spend a higher than average portion of it on health-related products and services.

Single males typically have no interest in spending any of their income on health care. Interactions with health care providers are minimal, and a high percentage do not have a personal physician. Single males constitute a significant share of the population that has access to employer-sponsored health care coverage but turns it down. Collectively, single households under the age of sixty-five comprise about one-fourth of all households and earn 18 percent of total household income.

Married Couples Without Children

Just over 18 percent of American households are composed of married couples under sixty-five without children. This market segment includes younger couples who have not yet started a family as well as older couples whose children are grown. Two incomes are the norm for this segment. Among the younger group both spouses often work and have access to health insurance through their employers. Those in the second group, the "empty nesters," are often at their peak earning capacity by the time the kids are gone. The family that no longer has children at home is typically the most attractive market for financial services firms. This group also has access to health care coverage through their employers.

Married couples without children control about 29 percent of household income—proportionately much higher than their numbers. Married couples without children have the largest proportion of their numbers in the highest income categories compared with other consumer market segments. Over one-third have high incomes, and another 58 percent have middle incomes.

The empty nesters in this segment are often astute and avid consumers of health care services. Expectations are high, and needs and wants are growing as many experience their first heart attack or opt for a face-lift to take away years from their appearance. This is the prime market for cosmetic surgery and the group that plastic surgeons pamper.

In the households of this segment the woman makes the major health-related decisions and directs health care consumption. However, men in this segment are showing more interest in health-related matters. A visit to any health club will confirm the interest of men in their physical condition.

Seniors

Although there is a wide variation in the subgroups that exist in this market segment, we limit our discussion to two: the healthy and the frail. Elderly households represent 18 percent of all U.S. households but earn about 10 percent of household income. However, because the entire group has access to Medicare, personal income is a less important market factor than in any of the other segments. Many lower-income seniors also participate in Medicaid, and the remainder typically have a supplemental insurance policy (Medigap) or participate in a Medicare risk plan (HMO).

The majority of senior households are in middle-income categories. Income distribution falls sharply as age increases beyond sixty-five. Likewise, the likelihood of living alone accelerates with age. Not surprisingly, frailty correlates with age and, to a lesser extent, income and household status. Approximately 4 percent of households in the country, or nearly 25 percent of senior households, can be classified as frail elderly, that is, needing assistance with the normal activities of daily living, such as meal preparation, bathing, dressing, and taking medications. This is the segment who are the highest consumers of health care services.

The other 75 percent of senior households are also large consumers of health care services, with increasing knowledge about health care. Influenced by their well-educated and demanding adult children, many are becoming active participants in their health care decisions and have lowered the pedestal on which physicians have traditionally been placed. (A few have removed the pedestal altogether!) They are conscious of what it takes to lead a healthy lifestyle, and although they realize they may not stay healthy forever, they are anxious to preserve their health and independence.

Market Segments: Summary

Each of the six market segments (married couples with children, single-parent families, singles under sixty-five, married couples without children, healthy seniors, and the frail elderly) has subgroups of sophisticated health care consumers with the financial resources to purchase what they want. Figure 7.4 shows our estimates of the proportion of Americans who are in the lead in terms of driving health care. The baby boomers and seniors are the biggest segments of Americans who combine a growing interest in health care with the ability to pay.

Other Factors Changing the Face of America

Although age and income are the key determinants of how individuals and families interact with the health care system, educational attainment, cultural diversity, and where people live are also important.

Education

Americans are increasingly better educated, with more disposable income and a higher net worth. These trends are occurring across all age groups. Educational levels continue to climb for the population overall. For example, in 1983 less than 18 percent of the noninstitutionalized adult population had completed four or more years of college. By 1998 the percentage was up to 24 percent. Real incomes have also gained over this period. Between 1993 and 1996 median household income increased by 6.8 percent on an inflation-adjusted basis (McNeil, 1998).

Why is this significant from a health care perspective? Regardless of age, two factors—income and education—are highly correlated with health status. A study by the Centers for Disease Control (CDC) concluded that for "almost all health indicators considered, each increase in either income or education increased the likelihood of being in good health" (U.S. Department of Health and Human Services, 1999, p. 2). Elaborating on this finding, the report noted that the greatest reduction in cigarette smoking between

Figure 7.4. Proportion of Households Most Interested in Health Care and with Above-Average Purchasing Power, 1996 and 2000.

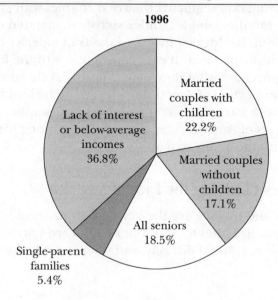

1996

Married couples with children
22.2%

Lack of interest or below-average incomes
36.8%

Married couples without children
17.1%

All seniors
18.5%

Single-parent families
5.4%

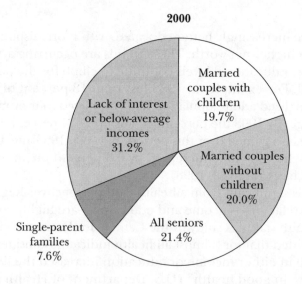

2000

Married couples with children
19.7%

Lack of interest or below-average incomes
31.2%

Married couples without children
20.0%

All seniors
21.4%

Single-parent families
7.6%

1974 and 1995 occurred among well-educated adults over twenty-five. Although this is good news for the ever larger proportion of people who are more highly educated and earn good incomes, the findings are discouraging for the less fortunate. Less well educated adults have higher death rates for all major causes of death, including chronic diseases, communicable diseases, and injuries.

Cultural Diversity

The United States, with its long tradition of immigrant populations, has always been a culturally and ethnically diverse country. Despite a more restrictive immigration policy than in the past, the tendency to become even more culturally heterogeneous is accelerating. Figure 7.5 depicts the racial and ethnic composition of the United States in 1990 and 2000 and projections for 2005. By 2010 minorities will make up 32 percent of the population, compared with 26 percent in 1990. The largest gains are expected among the Hispanic population, which will comprise nearly 13 percent of Americans in 2005.

When it comes to health status indicators, blacks and Hispanics nearly always rank below their white counterparts. Much of this is attributable to lower incomes and education. Based on the CDC report, over one-fifth of poor black children have high levels of toxins in their blood due to exposure to lead-based paint and other adverse environmental factors. Infants born to mothers who did not finish high school were about 50 percent more likely to be of low birth weight than infants whose mothers finished college (U.S. Department of Health and Human Services, 1999). Further evidence suggests that discrimination exists in how the medical profession deals with minorities. For example, a black woman is 60 percent less likely to be referred for a cardiac catheterization than a white woman with the same health history ("Health Care," 1999).

What are the implications of these cultural differences for health care providers? First, it is critical that health care be delivered in ways that are culturally appropriate. Education and outreach are essential to modify unhealthy behaviors of those who do not have access to, or who feel disenfranchised from, the health care system. It would also help to have more diversity among individuals delivering the care. Although women have made great strides in increasing

Figure 7.5. Racial and Ethnic Composition of the United States, 1990, 2000, and 2005.

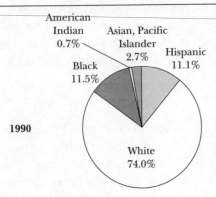

American Indian 0.7%
Asian, Pacific Islander 2.7%
Hispanic 11.1%
Black 11.5%
1990
White 74.0%

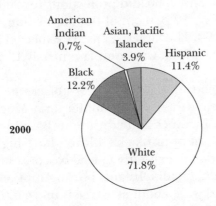

American Indian 0.7%
Asian, Pacific Islander 3.9%
Hispanic 11.4%
Black 12.2%
2000
White 71.8%

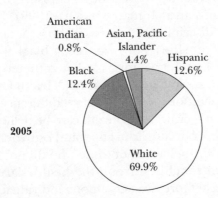

American Indian 0.8%
Asian, Pacific Islander 4.4%
Hispanic 12.6%
Black 12.4%
2005
White 69.9%

Source: "Health Care," 1999.

their representation in medical schools throughout the country, the same is not true for ethnic minorities. For example, Hispanics make up less than 3 percent of American doctors yet constitute 9 percent of the population ("Health Care," 1999).

Urban Versus Rural

Geographical dispersion of the population is also a factor in the changing face of America. Suburban areas continue to gain population at the expense of inner cities, and metropolitan areas continue to attract residents from rural America. The migration toward the South and West, and away from the Midwest and Northeast, has slowed in recent years but has not abated.

Rural areas have disproportionately more elderly and more lower-income households. At a retreat for a small rural hospital in Kansas, a board member commented, "We have fewer children in first grade this year than any other time in the last twenty-six years I've lived here." The challenge in rural areas is sustaining a viable health care system in light of a declining and aging population. Interestingly, rural residents use health care services less than their urban counterparts. A by-product of the migration from rural to urban areas, therefore, is accelerated health care spending. Residents of rural areas tend to be more self-reliant and are more conservative in using health care services. There are also fewer physicians conveniently available in rural areas.

One indicator of this phenomenon is Medicare's AAPCC rates. AAPCC rates reflect the average Medicare expenditures on a per capita basis for residents of a particular county regardless of where they receive care. So, for example, if seventy-five-year-old Mary living in Pratt, Kansas, travels to Wichita for heart surgery, dollars spent in Wichita are tracked back to her hometown. Therefore AAPCC data are a useful measure of regional health care utilization and spending.

A significant component of lower utilization in rural areas is the lack of access to specialized health services. Rural residents routinely go to a primary care physician or a physician's assistant rather than self-referring to a specialist. Rural residents also have more realistic expectations of the health care system. Farmers in Kansas, who see life, death, and disease every day on their farms and ranches, are more likely to accept the fact that the medical profession cannot cure everything and that "heroic" medical efforts are unwarranted. This more fatalistic view of the world can also be damaging to health status. One doctor practicing medicine in rural Maine indicated that some patients would not come to his second-story office in town because of the stairs. They preferred to see him at his satellite clinic in their own community. Whereas this would be understandable if he were talking about the elderly, he was actually referring to some of his patients who were around forty years old and just accepted their shortness of breath and fatigued muscles as a sign of age! "These folks in rural areas just don't know any better. They don't know that their lifestyle is what's responsible for their poor health status," he explained.

Regional Differences

Major regional variations exist in how health care is practiced; these variations, in turn, affect consumer perceptions and expectations. For example, in his research on regional variation Dr. John Wennberg and his colleagues (Dartmouth Medical School, 1996) note that the elderly on the East Coast, especially those living in major cities like Miami and New York, are more likely to spend their last days in an intensive care unit than elderly living on the West Coast. The litany of regional differences goes on and on. These variations have a dramatic impact on health care costs and influence consumer expectations. As time goes by and people become ever more migratory, consumers are likely to exert more influence over these wide variations in treatment practices. But this will take time.

Future Shifts in Demographics and Chronic Diseases

How are the market segments likely to evolve in the future? Life expectancies and the progression of chronic diseases will have enormous impact on the demand for health care services.

Life Expectancies

Life expectancies continue to climb as more people live longer. For example, individuals who reach 65 can expect to have another

17 years ahead of them. The number of years beyond 65 quickly expands as the baby boomers move up into these age ranks. A woman reaching 65 in 2020 can expect to live to be 86.5, or 2.6 more years than the same woman who turned 65 in 1990. In fact, as Deets (1999) notes, over half of all people who have ever lived to be 65 are alive today.

The impact of longer life expectancies comes at a time when the largest age cohort in our society will be moving into the ranks of Americans 65 and over, thus amplifying what is already an enormous demographic event. The baby boom generation, born between 1946 and 1964, begins to reach 65 in 2011, and the numbers go up from there. By 2030 individuals over 65 will constitute 20 percent of the population, compared with 14 percent in 2000.

Chronic Conditions

Longer life expectancies are not all good news. Although longer life might be hailed as a sign of progress, a portion of these extended years may not be pleasant. Estimates indicate that as many as 5.3 years of life after 65 will be unhealthy (American Association for World Health, 1999). Debilitating chronic conditions are not limited to the elderly. A Robert Wood Johnson report, *Chronic Care in America: A 21st Century Challenge,* sheds light on the prevalence and high cost of chronic care (see "Chronic Care in America," 1996). Approximately one hundred million Americans have one or more chronic conditions. The elderly constitute one-fourth of those with chronic illnesses. Many elderly also suffer from multiple chronic conditions. Table 7.1 profiles the top ten chronic illnesses among older Americans and compares them to the leading causes of death among this population.

Although an increasing number of people successfully cope with chronic conditions, for others chronic ailments can be debilitating. So as we look at the changing face of America, it is important to note that the proportion of the population suffering from chronic diseases is increasing. Between 1987 and 1993 the number of individuals with a chronic disabling condition grew 20 percent to 27 million. By 2020 chronic conditions will affect 134 million, with 39 million experiencing disabling limitations. These trends toward increasing numbers of Americans with chronic

Table 7.1. Top Ten Health Problems of Older Americans.

Top Ten Chronic Conditions	Top Ten Causes of Death
1. Arthritis	1. Diseases of the heart
2. High blood pressure	2. Malignant neoplasms (cancer)
3. Hearing impairment	3. Cerebrovascular diseases and stroke
4. Diseases of the heart	
5. Cataracts	4. Chronic obstructive pulmonary diseases, emphysema
6. Limb deformities or impairments	
7. Chronic sinusitis	5. Pneumonia and influenza
8. Diabetes	6. Diabetes mellitus
9. Tinnitus (ringing in the ears)	7. Unintentional injuries
10. Visual impairment	8. Alzheimer's disease
	9. Kidney disease
	10. Blood stream infections

Source: American Association for World Health, 1999, p. 11.

health conditions have significant implications for health care providers, Medicare, Medicaid, health plans, and disease management companies.

Baby Boomers as a Market Force

Increasingly educated, empowered, and wealthy consumers will change the shape of health care delivery. And baby boomers do not have to wait until they reach their senior years or develop chronic conditions; they are a potent force today. In the year 2000 baby boomers, representing 30 percent of the population, were between the ages of thirty-five and fifty-four. Many are caring for aging parents as well as growing children (U.S. Department of Commerce, Bureau of the Census, 1996). They are taking better care of themselves and spending huge amounts of money to deter or mitigate the aging process. They have spawned whole new fields of work: Who but a professional athlete had a personal trainer ten years ago? One marketer observes, "From jogging to plastic surgery, from vegetarian diets to Viagra, they are fighting to preserve their youth and defy the effects of gravity" (Howgill, 1998, p. 40).

Compared with their parents, baby boomers are far more demanding of the health care system and have higher expectations. Press, Ganey Associates, a firm that tracks patient satisfaction levels in many hospitals, reports that baby boomers give lower marks on all counts, from food quality to the decor of the hospital and the level of attention and service they receive (Bellandi, 1998). As one marketer put it, "The hallmark of the generation is that it will protest for what it believes and demands whatever it wants" (Howgill, 1998, p. 40). Baby boomers are much less likely to be passive recipients of medical care and more likely to be active consumers of health services (Institute for the Future, 1998).

What Lies Ahead?

As we look at the changing face of America as it relates to health care, we see that people are becoming older, wealthier, better informed, more diverse, and more demanding. Baby boomers will lead this trend, both as consumers themselves and as caregivers for their aging parents. A more culturally diverse population will increasingly challenge traditional relationships and approaches.

The explosion of access to information (discussed in Chapter Eight) and the continued migratory nature of Americans will lead to a reduction in regional variation. However, access to health-related information will be uneven. Less well educated, lower-income individuals will continue to rely on traditional sources of information while their more educated, higher-income counterparts will have a vast array of information available to them.

For the majority, differences in whether they are rural or urban consumers, Californians or New Yorkers, will tend to diminish in importance over time. Hopefully, differences in access to health care based on race and ethnicity will also disappear, but we are less confident of this outcome in the absence of a payment mechanism for the uninsured.

Chapter Eight

The Meaning of the Internet and Information Technology

The analogy I use is electricity. You've got to go a long way back in history to find something that was equally profound in its impact, not just on business but on society.
KIM B. CLARK, DEAN OF HARVARD BUSINESS SCHOOL,
Harvard Magazine, May–June 1999

Of all the factors affecting health care in the new millennium, the unprecedented role of the Internet and the development of clinical information systems have to rate among the most important. This chapter includes an overview of the potential for the Internet to alter consumer and provider behavior. We also report on clinical information systems development and the connection of these systems with clinical guidelines and outcomes measurement. Our purpose is to develop insights about the impact of the Internet and IT on the health care financing and delivery systems of the future. This chapter is closely related to Chapter Nine, which reviews genetic research, new drugs, and likely advances in medical technology. These two chapters add up to a picture of rapid innovation and change in store for health care over the next five years.

Referring to the revolutionary impact of the Internet, Andrew Grove, chairman of Intel, puts it this way: "We are in a period of major change that is dictated by the fact that consumers of health care services are ahead of the profession in their embrace of electronic means of getting information, participating in support groups, handling transactions and communicating. And this is likely to drive the acceptance of these techniques throughout the medical profession" (Intel Corp., 1998). In assessing the importance of information in health care, Leland Kaiser, a well-known health care futurist, says, "Information is power. Some people think of healthcare as a service industry; I think of it as an information-based enterprise" (interview, Mar. 31, 1999).

Exhibit 8.1 summarizes the growth and anticipated impacts of the Internet.

The Potential of the Internet to Influence Health Care

Leland Kaiser believes the Internet is already revolutionizing the way people get their health care information and the decisions they make. "Beyond just getting access to state-of-art medical information," Kaiser said, "consumers are acting upon this new information. The sophistication of the chat boxes, or users' groups, is unbelievable. Also, with clinical guidelines now readily available, patients have access to information on how they should manage many of their own diseases or ailments of a family member" (interview, Mar. 31, 1999). Kaiser went on to say that he sees the role of

Exhibit 8.1. Highlights in the Internet and Information Technology.

- The Internet will become the information source on medical advice for physicians and consumers around the world.
- The quality of health information on Web sites will improve; a few trustworthy and highly credible sites will emerge.
- Telehealth will facilitate the monitoring and delivery of additional health services to individuals in their homes.
- There will be an immense increase in e-mail communications between patients and physicians.
- Telemedicine as we know it today will be replaced by high-speed Internet-based transmission of clinical information.
- Telemedicine will be used to link U.S. medical groups with hospitals in many foreign countries and will lead to new business opportunities.
- The electronic medical record and other clinical databases will provide physicians and analysts tremendous opportunities to measure and improve clinical outcomes.

physicians changing in this new consumer-driven system where patients have ready access to the Internet: "Especially for chronic diseases, physicians will be coaches or trusted advisors. Sure, they will continue to prescribe medication and perform other traditional functions. However, they have lost the mystery of 'black box' medicine; patients may know as much about their own illnesses as their doctors."

We estimate that half of all U.S. households have at least one personal computer (PC) and that most of these households are connected to the Internet and have e-mail. With the price of PCs dropping dramatically and connection and processing speeds growing exponentially (note, for example, the competition between cable television firms and telephone companies to see who can deliver the best bandwidth and the fastest connections), by 2005 Internet access and use in the United States will reach the point where almost every household will have access to this communication technology. And then there is the rest of the world— also making its way on-line. Potential consumer uses of the Internet for health care are shown in Figure 8.1.

Use of E-Mail in Health Care

E-mail has tremendous untapped potential, particularly for patient-to-physician communication. Andrew Grove of Intel noted that although the majority of doctors use e-mail to communicate with other doctors, an almost negligible portion of physicians use e-mail to communicate with patients. "This is very, very strange to me," Grove remarked. At Intel all seventy thousand employees have e-mail and prefer it to the telephone and other means of communication by a factor of ten to one, but as Grove said (Intel Corp., 1998):

> It is puzzling that this same phenomenon would not be at work in the medical world, in the health care world, and particularly when you consider that another layer of utility comes from conducting garden-variety, routine transactions, ordering medicines, filling prescriptions, asking routine questions, things that are kind of the housekeeping of a company—the fundamental work of medicine. . . . Increasingly, the water is surrounding the castle here. And it is happening on over-the-counter areas, where it is

Figure 8.1. Growing Uses of the Internet in Health Care for Consumers.

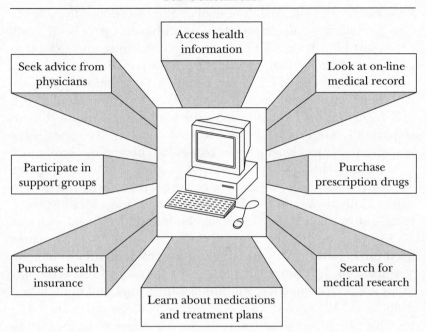

Access health
information

Seek advice from
physicians

Look at on-line
medical record

Participate in
support groups

Purchase
prescription drugs

Purchase health
insurance

Search for
medical research

Learn about medications
and treatment plans

unregulated, it is happening in alternative medicine areas, it is happening in nutritional supplements and all of that stuff. Sites that can fulfill these transaction requirements proliferate.

Research on Use of Patient-Physician E-Mail

David Stern described a research project being conducted at the University of Michigan (Intel Corp., 1998). The purpose of the study was to evaluate the content and efficiency of patient-physician e-mail as well as the satisfaction of the patients and physicians with their e-mail communication. Stern summarized the results: "I think e-mail like this is a very powerful tool," he said. "If we can learn to manage it well and fit it into the work flow of physicians and of patients—even though physicians and patients have some concerns about using e-mail—patients are really going to latch onto it."

One Physician's Perspective on E-mail

In assessing the potential for e-mail communication with patients, one physician-administrator told us, "I haven't practiced in six years, but I know that if I came in every morning and I saw that there were fifteen e-mail messages from my patients, I would freak out. I already receive fifty to sixty e-mails a day from other doctors, and there is voice mail on top of that. Then you have regular mail and information from the lab and hospital. Someone has to respond to all of this, but how?" He went on to say, "However, there are advantages to e-mail when it comes to patients. You have more latitude in deciding when to respond as compared with a message to return a patient's call and no background on why the person called. The answer to this increased flow of messages has to be some sort of triage system involving the staff of the doctor's office." This physician-administrator concluded, "It really doesn't matter what physicians think; patients are going to demand e-mail communications. It is more convenient for them, and this is the way many are accustomed to communicating at work and in their personal lives." We agree with this assessment. Consumers are going to drive physicians to more frequent use of e-mail in their communications with patients.

Another Viewpoint on E-Mail

Eugenia Marcus, a pediatrician in Newton, Massachusetts, says that with e-mail patients can send messages whenever they think about it and that she can respond at her convenience. "I don't have to worry about whether I'm calling when they're between work and home, and there's no phone tag," she says (Stevens, 1998, p. 24). Marcus is using e-mail to broadcast announcements like the availability of flu shots and was considering an electronic newsletter to patients. This approach would eliminate the cost of paper, printing, and mailing. Although e-mail reaches only a minority of patients, she notes that the number of patients with e-mail access is growing rapidly. "Over the past three months," Marcus says, "I've noticed a quantum leap in the number of patients who have e-mail either at home or at work" (p. 26).

The Potential of E-Mail for Physician-to-Patient Communication

Mark Levine, associate medical director of the Colorado Foundation for Medical Care, believes that e-mail has more potential for physicians communicating with patients than the other way around: "I can see e-mail being used to communicate test results and follow-up information for use by the patient," he told us. "E-mail is a superior way to communicate much of this information."

Health Plan–Physician E-Mail

Levine also believes that one of the best potential applications of e-mail is between physicians and health plans. In Levine's opinion, "This could speed up approvals and other information flow, and not be as disruptive as the constant stream of phone calls." The types of information that could effectively flow through e-mail include patient eligibility, referrals, preauthorizations, guidelines, medical management information, and clinical results.

Improving the Quality of Health Information on the Web

In 1999 there were over fifteen thousand Web sites providing health information, with the number growing daily. "Almost half of all consumers have used the Internet for health information in the last 12 months," Dr. Grove said (Intel Corp., 1998).

Evaluating the Information

One information expert, acknowledging that consumers have access to a huge amount of information on the Internet, asked a pertinent question: How are they supposed to sort through it? As this expert observed, "There's a lot of garbage out there." The need to filter Internet-based data is already leading to new business opportunities. For example, two Denver physicians established ProMedica, a company that helps consumers sift through a pile of information before they make any medical decisions or take the material with them to see their physicians. According to Bob Truckner, cofounder of the new firm, "Doctors are complaining people are coming with 30 pages from the Internet, but with no scientific validity." Truckner explains, "Our strong point is you're handing the physician something he understands" (Hubler, 1999, p. J4).

Whether or not ProMedica is successful, start-up ventures of this type are harbingers of the future use of Internet-based medical information. Identifying medical information on the Internet and assessing its value can be expected to take on ever greater importance in the years ahead. The criticism that Internet-based medical information is of uneven quality will continue to be valid, but there will be resources available to scrutinize and assess the data. We anticipate that many of the most reputable U.S. health care organizations, including a number of medical schools, will see this as a business opportunity and be active in this arena. We already have the Harvard and Mayo health newsletters, among many others.

Big Information Technology Players Invest Heavily in Health Care

It was a routine announcement: two Internet-based start-up companies, WebMD and Healtheon, were merging. Healtheon was a Silicon Valley company specializing in medical transaction processing. WebMD was an Atlanta company that operated Web sites tailored to consumers and professionals. Prior to the merger announcement the two companies had 1998 revenues of less than $50 million. The value of the merger was an astounding $9.84 billion (Clark, 1999, p. B6). Here was the attention grabber: Microsoft, Intel, and Excite had become investors in the combined company. The *Wall Street Journal* article reported, "The merger creates the most potent Internet company offering services and information for doctors, patients and other healthcare players" (p. B6). Microsoft contributed $250 million in equity, and the other investors added over $100 million more to the merged company. According to a Microsoft executive, "Bringing Healtheon and WebMD together creates an environment where you can really empower consumers, and at the same time help reduce waste in the healthcare system" (p. B6).

Delivery of Health Care Through Telehealth

Telehealth is sometimes defined as the remote delivery of any kind of care. Regarding the potential growth of telehealth, the Institute for the Future discusses "the amazing recent discovery in American health care that the care of sick people is expensive, and the more you can do to keep them healthy, the less money they'll cost" (Institute for the Future, 1999, p. 2). This comment suggests what the consumer-driven health care system of the future must deliver.

Remote care depends on the development of new types of biosensors that will be temporarily attached to, or even permanently implanted in, patients in order to record clinical information such as blood sugar, heart rate, and so on, alert a human if necessary, and make adjustments in medication. As one prediction describes it, "The patient will be automatically monitored as the sensors communicate back to the provider organization over networks, including the Internet. Better outcomes with few hospital days and happier patients and payers are the promise" (Institute for the Future, 1999, p. 5).

Dr. John Koster, CEO, Washington, Providence Health System, anticipates something similar: "In the future consumers will have home testing devices that connect to providers via the Internet," he told us. "This will allow real-time, cost-effective, and convenient management of certain health problems. Certain pharmaceutical and device manufacturers may, over time, find that home testing and monitoring via the Internet will give them *direct access* to patients, the end consumers of the products. This will accelerate the 'disintermediation' of traditional providers." Dr. Mark Levine of HealthCare Colorado agrees and also sees the potential for personalized disease management for patients. "The Internet and e-mail," he said, "tremendously increase the feasibility of directing disease management to a patient on a one-on-one basis."

The Institute for the Future (1999, p. 5) sums it up this way: "Overall, the future of the Internet in medical care is that of a venue for real care management of many varied types, mostly achieved remotely and with a minimum of human intervention. A combination of open networks, transaction standards, and sensor technologies will provide the opportunity to get us there. The real challenge will be for all of us in American health care to develop the financial incentives and human and organizational solutions to get us there in ten years, rather than thirty."

We agree; the organizational and financial challenges required to implement the kind of future described here are more challenging than the technological issues. At the same time we believe that consumers will drive these kinds of changes and that physicians, hospitals, and other providers will respond. And as evidenced by the merger of Healtheon and WebMD (and the investment of millions of dollars by Microsoft, Intel, and Excite), it will not take ten years. Many of the kinds of changes and much of the potential discussed in the preceding paragraphs will become reality during the first five years of the new millennium.

Telemedicine

Generally speaking, telemedicine involves sending medical data between two locations electronically, through videoconferencing, sound, digitized patient records, and high-resolution images, such as X rays. In traditional telemedicine, information is sent over high-speed telephone lines or by satellite.

Types of Telemedicine Services

There are at least four uses of telemedicine (Institute for the Future, 1999):

- *Consultation:* direct physician-patient interactions, such as psychiatric consultations, wound checks, care for those in correctional institutions, or analysis of dermatological symptoms that can be done using videoconference facilities
- *Diagnosis:* remote reading of digitized radiology images, such as MRIs or X rays, or analysis of pathology images
- *Education:* Continuing medical education classes and transmission of grand rounds or surgery live to a remote but interactive audience
- *Invasive treatment:* remote treatment, including the use of image-guided surgery systems (this is still in the experimental phase)

Regarding the last point, invasive treatment using telemedicine, the potential for U.S. physicians and health care providers to expand around the world is mind boggling. Following is one example that may be the first of many.

Mayo Clinic and Middle East Hospitals Use Telemedicine

The Mayo Clinic opened a telemedicine service at the Abu Dhabi–Al Mafraq Hospital system in the United Arab Emigrates. According to an article that describes the service (Cochrane, 1999b, p. 15), "The technology linking this two-hospital system with the Mayo Clinic enables both hospitals to exchange digitized data and high-resolution, diagnostic video images. Al Mafraq Hospital is also buying an electronic medical records system which will make it possible to establish physician-to-physician contact via the telemedicine link." The initial telemedicine consultations focus on cardiovascular diseases. "But the scope will be broadened to cover neurosurgery, orthopedics, dermatology, oncology and other disciplines" (p. 15).

Cochrane concludes, "As yet, neither telemedicine nor international business have added much to the bottom lines of most American hospital systems who have tried it. But, it's clear that even now, the technology exists to create a 'global medical village' in the future" (p. 15). We agree with Cochrane—the global potential for expansion of medical services originating in the United States is tremendous. Health care could become one of our major export industries (this is discussed further in scenarios 3 and 4 in Chapter Thirteen).

Growth of Telemedicine

Future short-term growth of traditional telemedicine is almost certain if several critical barriers can be reduced or eliminated. These include the decision of many insurance companies not to reimburse physicians and hospitals for this type of service, physician resistance to the technology, concern over the impact of telemedicine on traditional referral patterns, and the licensing of medical professionals across state lines (for example, a primary care physician in a hospital in western Kansas seeking advice from a specialist in Denver who is not licensed in Kansas).

It appears that the barriers to the international use of telemedicine may be substantially less complicated than those experienced in the United States. Furthermore, telemedicine applications involving large and prestigious medical groups, like the Mayo

Clinic and its partners in the Middle East, is almost certain to stimulate increased use of telemedicine in the U.S. marketplace.

Will the Internet Replace Telemedicine?

There are a number of experts who believe the Internet will replace telemedicine in the first five years of the twenty-first century. Henry Lowe of the University of Pittsburgh School of Medicine believes the uniqueness of telemedicine will soon pass. "Telemedicine," he predicts, "will become integrated with the Internet. Internet-based healthcare is imminent."

Lowe anticipates a paradigm shift in health care. "As healthcare becomes more electronic, it will become more patient centered." This will happen partly because we are moving into the era of broadband technology. He envisions a transition to a broadband Internet-based "multimedia" electronic medical record (EMR). "At this point," according to Lowe, "telemedicine will disappear." In other words the Internet will be capable of transmitting all types of data and images, including video, and there will be no need for telemedicine as we know it today.

Dr. John Silva of the Defense Advanced Research Projects Agency observes that telemedicine had to buy its own pathways and that, for this reason, it will not survive in the long run. Silva predicts that because of the Internet and the increased availability of broadband access, "We will soon have an order of magnitude increase in the ability to share information."

We agree with Lowe and Silva in their conclusion that the Internet will soon change telemedicine as we know it today. The relatively high cost of telemedicine, for such items as equipment and access, and limitations on the use of telemedicine suggest the Internet will be a superior method of delivering the types of services telemedicine has traditionally provided.

Information Technology in Health Care

By the mid-1980s there were a dozen companies striving to create an automated medical record. However, most of the efforts were not successful, and only one of the original twelve survived. Efforts to create integrated health care systems in the late 1980s and early

1990s jump-started investment in health care IT and led to the current high level of interest in the field.

Although the health care industry continues to lag in terms of IT investment, it is not uncommon for a midsize hospital and associated medical group to invest $2 to $3 million a year in clinical and management information system development. Larger systems, like the Marshfield Clinic and Geisinger, continue to invest substantially more.

Information Technology: What Are We Talking About?

There continues to be interest in clinical information systems for medical groups, hospitals (most commonly for labs, radiology, and pharmacy), and health plans. Many of these types of single-purpose systems can be purchased from any of hundreds of vendors. Walk through the exhibit halls at the annual meetings of the Medical Group Management Association, Healthcare Information and Management Systems Society (HIMSS), or the Healthcare Financial Management Association, and you get an idea of the multitude of IT alternatives available.

Claims Data

Health plans have used their claims data to build large databases. One hospital CEO told us, "Some of our more sophisticated health plan customers know more about us and our physicians than we know about ourselves." With the consolidation of health plans, we expect these kinds of information systems to become increasingly important in assessing inappropriate and unnecessary care and identifying preferred provider groups and physicians.

Integrated Information Systems

One of the biggest challenges is the integration of physician and hospital clinical databases. Most of the large integrated health care organizations (for example, Carle Clinic in Illinois, Intermountain Health Care in Utah) are investing in these types of integrated information systems.

There are several aspects to these more complex systems. They all include the EMR for both hospital and outpatient services, including prescriptions. They usually incorporate laboratory and imaging results. Most of these types of clinical information systems also include clinical guidelines and a database to measure outcomes. In a sense these information systems are designed to provide the feedback for continuously improving clinical processes.

Information Technology, Continuous Quality Improvement, and Outcomes

The relationship between clinical information, CQI, and outcomes measurement is illustrated in Figure 8.2. Although it is normal to think of outcomes data being used primarily to impress payers, most large provider systems use this information to close the loop in their quality improvement processes. It is the feedback mechanism.

On the issue of outcomes measurement Richard Huber, former chairman, CEO, and president of Aetna, has this to say regarding IT: "Without being disrespectful, I consider the U.S. healthcare delivery system the largest cottage industry in the world. There are virtually no performance measurements and no standards. We all know the studies about these incredible variances in the instances of certain procedures across the population, which there is no

Figure 8.2. Reducing Clinical Variation.

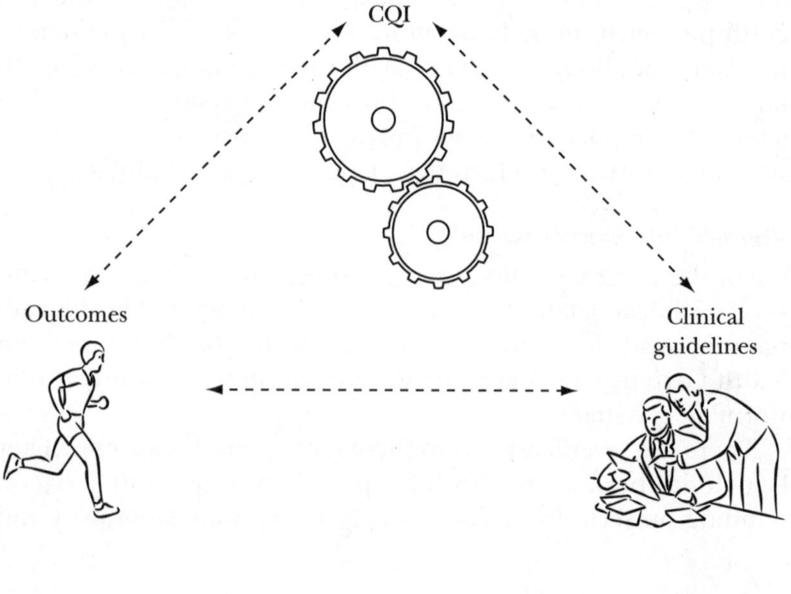

rational way to explain. . . . Trying to measure performance, to measure outcomes, and to bring some degree of standardization to this system is the next revolution in health care" ("The Future of Health Care," 1999, p. 45).

We have been hearing about efforts to measure and report outcomes for the past decade, and the results to date have not been impressive. But we agree with Huber that more meaningful outcomes measurement is coming, probably toward the end of the five-year period we are most concerned about in this book, and it will be part of the revolution in health care. Advances in IT will facilitate this revolution.

Electronic Medical Records

We have visited many more hospitals and medical groups that are investing in the development of the EMR than those that could demonstrate a full-scale, operating system. However, operational clinical information systems do exist. In 1997, for example, one of the authors witnessed a primary care physician at one of the Marshfield Clinic's regional centers using such a system. He said, "It is especially valuable in keeping track of prescriptions for elderly patients who see a number of our specialists, or for those who use an [emergency room] in another facility and then come to me for additional care." In 1998 Kaiser Permanente also installed such a system in its fifteen Denver area medical offices. Although reported to be slow, the system is operational.

Patient Access to Medical Records

There are a number of new ventures being developed that have as their focus making the EMR accessible to patients. For example, Ikenna Okezie, one of the first two people to pursue a joint degree in business and medicine from Harvard, has formulated a business plan for AccessMED, a health care IT company that would give patients on-line access to their medical records. "Physicians don't always share enough information about a patient's status and treatment, which makes many patients anxious at a time when they already feel a lack of control," explains Okezie (Ross, 1999, p. 31). AccessMED would be available to patients through their HMOs and would link them on-line with their lab results, diagnoses, medications, and other relevant information. "We hope to prove that patients will comply more readily with treatment regimens when they understand them better" (p. 31).

The *Wall Street Journal* reports that consumers may soon be deluged with options for maintaining their medical records on the Internet: "Some services in the pipeline, like the tentatively named AboutMyHealth.net from MedicaLogic Inc., Hillsboro, Ore., will primarily be made available to patients through their doctors, who will maintain the data. Others, like PersonalMD.com, an offshoot of closely held NeoTrax Corp., Pleasanton, Calif., plan to work with doctors and health systems but are initially recruiting consumers directly" (Carrns, 1999, p. B1). As the article also explains, "A similar offering is in the works from drkoop.com Inc., the Austin, Texas, Internet health company founded by former U.S. surgeon general C. Everett Koop. The patient is responsible for entering and maintaining the data, and deciding who gets access. 'If you wait for your doctor to do it, it will never happen,' says Donald Hackett, chief executive of drkoop.com" (p. B1).

Physicians' Views on Clinical Information Systems

Steven S. Lazarus, a health care information systems consultant, says that physicians want a clinical information system with these characteristics (Lazarus, 1999):

- Speed—the ability to support or increase current production
- Reasonably short training time
- Mobility
- System functionality that is the same in offices and hospitals
- Full integration with the billing system
- Integrated tools for disease management and managed care administrative requirements
- Reliability
- Affordability

Lazarus told us, "Getting physicians to accept and use a clinical information system remains one of the biggest barriers. However, as we have more case studies of organizations that have successfully implemented these types of systems, it will help immensely in selling physicians on the value of this way of doing business." We believe that such case studies will become widely available in the next two or three years.

Lazarus identifies eight potential benefits of a fully implemented EMR (1999):

1. Records would be accessible from multiple sites.
2. Multiple providers could access a single record simultaneously.
3. Increased productivity and patient throughput could be achieved.
4. There could be decision support (especially for avoiding adverse drug reactions), fewer duplicate and unnecessary tests, and intervention as a part of disease management efforts.
5. Compliance with Medicare and payer requirements could be ensured by linking documentation and billing.
6. Significant reductions could be made in medical records staff and transcription staff.
7. Departmental and other duplicative paper records could be eliminated.
8. Best practice protocols could be developed, and the quality of care could be improved.

Will these benefits be realized and, if so, when? We know of several large integrated systems that are just beginning to realize these kinds of benefits, and we anticipate that in the next five years many more organizations will reap the rewards of their investment in clinical IT.

Information Technology and Consumers

We remain convinced that once patients are exposed to the EMR, especially in the setting of a large integrated system where all of their records (such as primary care and specialist visits, hospitalizations, and test results) are accessible in one place, they will be extremely pleased with the results. In communities where there are two competing health care systems, one with a fully developed EMR and the other using paper records, it is not difficult to predict which system will be the winner at the dawn of the consumer movement.

Neal Patterson, chairman, president, and CEO of Cerner Corporation, one of the leading health care IT companies, says that IT is all about the "person." Speaking at the HIMSS annual conference held Feb. 23, 1999, Patterson explained, "No one wants to be a patient; we all want to be persons." He added, "Persons want a healthcare system that caters to their needs, not the physician's or hospital staff's needs. They want access when they need it. Personally I want a physician who knows me, my kids and my parents. This relates to advances in genomic research, and the fact that 75 percent of the diseases that people die from are in their genes. I don't know about you, but I want a healthcare system to focus on me."

Longitudinal Enterprise Databases

We first heard the term *longitudinal enterprise database* when visiting Intermountain Health Care (IHC) in Utah. It refers to the development of clinical databases on patients (outpatient and inpatient) over a long period of time so that studies of patient health status and the outcomes of medical procedures can be measured in more meaningful ways.

Al Pryor, an executive with IHC, said that the development of a longitudinal enterprise database at IHC required four major steps (Coddington, Chapman, and Pokoski, 1996):

1. *Compile a centralized master member index.* Pryor and others said that this is much more difficult than it would seem.
2. *Create the interface between hospitals and the longitudinal database.*
3. *Devise codes for information that will be input into the system.* Having information available in a coded format facilitates analysis and is critical for process improvement efforts.
4. *Build the decision support part of the system.* This is needed to activate the care process models (clinical guidelines). Pryor said, "These models are useless unless you can incorporate them into your computerized information system. Physicians won't use them unless they have immediate access" (p. 43).

Related to the last point, Pryor said that when you want to interact with physicians, you cannot have a system that slows them down.

"They already think they know the answers, and they usually do. However, we are trying to develop a more standardized approach and this is where the process models and the clinical information system fit in" (p. 43).

Based on our experience, the IHC effort, which has been ongoing for over twenty years, is more comprehensive than most information system initiatives in medical groups and hospitals. Part of this is due to IHC's strong emphasis on CQI and the need for data to facilitate that process. We expect larger health care systems, particularly those that have integrated physician and hospital care in a multispecialty setting, to continue to develop these types of longitudinal and enterprise-wide databases. Although developing these databases is expensive and time consuming, the results promise to be exciting.

A Health Plan Perspective

Health plans have in many respects been the pioneers in developing useful data on quality of care, utilization of physicians and hospitals, and costs. It appears that with the continued consolidation of health plans (discussed in more detail in Chapter Ten), these organizations will make massive investments in collecting and analyzing information, allowing them to improve the quality and cost-effectiveness of the care delivered by physicians and hospitals under contract with them.

In this regard John Kelly (1998), president of U.S. Quality Algorithms, Aetna U.S. Healthcare Inc., says he has learned that

- Effective managed care requires accurate, accessible, and automated administrative, financial, and clinical information
- Analysis of automated data on health plans, hospitals, physicians, and enrollees guides organization strategies, influences provider contracts and reimbursement, informs provider and enrollee education, and facilitates patient management
- Automated information is essential for effective and efficient quality, utilization, disease, and resource management
- Despite the limitations of available sources of automated data, thoughtful analysis and interpretation of available data allow automated information to be used effectively and responsibly

Reducing Errors in Drug Dosages: A Significant Payoff

As we enter an era when clinical information systems are beginning to show benefits, what are the payoffs? Steven Lazarus told us that the major benefits will be in improving the accuracy of prescriptions and reducing the chances for errors and duplicate dosages. According to Neal Patterson, there are huge errors in both prescriptions and compliance on the part of patients. As he pointed out at the 1999 HIMSS conference, "If you build the IT system and input the knowledge, you have the basis for intervention in these kinds of problems. This is where the payoff comes from IT."

Another speaker at the same conference noted that each year $20 billion worth of prescriptions are not filled. "With a properly-designed clinical information system," this speaker said, "the physician would at least know whether the prescription has been filled. This suggests that it would be in the interests of drug companies to get more active in developing and financing clinical information systems."

In support of the value of clinical IT in avoiding adverse drug events, Joseph Newhouse, director of Harvard's division of health policy research and education, says, "If you're a doctor at Brigham and Women's Hospital and you order a drug, you enter it into a computer. And if there's a problem with the dosage you ordered or an interaction with other medications, the computer's going to spit it back at you and the patient won't get the drug. We know that there are a non-trivial number of adverse drug events that could be prevented. This is one area where information technology can help" ("The Future of Health Care," 1999, p. 49).

All four of the authors have had either personal experiences with errors in prescription drugs or have had someone in their family with this type of experience. The mother of one author was receiving dosages of an addictive pain-killing drug from two different physicians. It took ten very painful days that included hallucinations, disorientation, and much screaming to get her off these drugs. The wife of another author was given the wrong prescription for her heart arrhythmia. Fortunately, she discovered the mistake before taking any of the pills! There are many more stories we could tell.

Information Technology and the Internet

We led off this chapter with a discussion of the impressive potential implications of the Internet for health care. But how does the Internet relate to clinical information systems development? According to several speakers at the 1999 HIMSS conference, the two are inextricably entwined.

The type of system that could pick up failures to have prescriptions filled would, in all likelihood, be Internet based and involve a variety of players, including physicians, patients, and pharmacists. The scheduling of visits to physicians' offices and accessing information from disease management programs are additional examples of possible uses of the Internet.

From a provider perspective the combination of health care IT and the Internet could facilitate collaboration among hospitals. It could be a tremendous asset for loosely knit managed care networks, such as IPAs and PHOs. It is already a reality for multispecialty clinics and integrated health care systems with multiple primary care sites.

Health Insurance Portability and Accountability Act

The Health Insurance Portability and Accountability Act (HIPAA), passed in 1996 but not yet fully implemented in 1999, has a role to play in the cost of health care IT and the speed of development. HIPAA calls for standard identifiers for providers, employers, and health plans and for security of patient data. The standards are applicable to all payers, not just Medicare and Medicaid.

Steven Lazarus says that implementation of HIPAA will bring down the setup and maintenance costs for electronic commerce between payers and providers and between medical groups and hospitals. "I believe," he told us, "that HIPAA standardization will have a profound effect on accelerating implementation of e-commerce in healthcare."

Implications of Advances in Health Care Information Systems: Summary

What are the future implications of the huge investment in health care information systems? We believe that the payoff will be profound; the question is *when*. Leland Kaiser told us he believes that within ten years most of the bugs will be worked out and community-wide medical records will be the norm. "It won't even be an issue; it will be an accomplished fact. Remember all of the questions about who would control automated teller machines and how they would be interconnected? Consumers prevailed and the banks got the job done."

Conclusions

What will the future bring in the way of new developments that will affect health care financing and delivery? It is difficult to say with precision, but based on the past we can be sure that the changes will be profound.

Here are the highlights of what can be expected over the next five years:

- With widespread ownership of PCs and broadband capability, the Internet will take over as *the* information source on medical advice for physicians and consumers around the world. The role of Internet-based support groups will be substantially greater than we could ever have anticipated.
- There will be an immense increase in e-mail communications between physicians and patients. Many routine matters— filling prescriptions, answering basic questions—will be handled via e-mail. In 2005 people will be asking, "Remember back when we used to go to the doctor's office for common ailments?" One of the unresolved issues, however, is how physicians will be paid for this type of communication.
- The EMR, along with longitudinal enterprise-wide databases, will provide physicians and analysts tremendous opportunities to measure clinical outcomes for use as feedback in quality improvement efforts and for reporting to the public. Patients will enjoy the convenience of computerized medical records when they go to a physician's office or hospital and are not required to provide the same information (age, allergies, prescriptions now being taken, insurance coverage, and so on) over and over again; patients will appreciate being recognized as "persons."

- Continuing emphasis on developing and applying clinical guidelines may not solve the problem of the disheartening amount of clinical variation in American medicine today, but it should put a dent in the amount of inappropriate and unnecessary care. As a result, quality of care will be improved.

Chapter Nine continues our discussion of biomedical research, new drugs, and advances in medical technology likely to affect health care during the first years of the new millennium.

Chapter Nine

The Impact of Genetic Research, New Drugs, and Advances in Medical Technology

For all the touting of a final genetic knockout of disease, there is no reason to expect such an event.

DANIEL CALLAHAN, *False Hopes: Why America's Quest for Perfect Health Is a Recipe for Failure,* Simon & Schuster, 1998

Not a day goes by that we do not read about advances in medical technology, new findings from genetic research, and drugs designed to improve quality of life and offer relief for those suffering from chronic diseases. One of the objectives of this chapter is to summarize research into genetics and its implications for the development of new drugs. The explosive growth of new drugs and medical technology are discussed along with the implications for consumers, physicians, and hospitals.

Before proceeding we should note that Daniel Callahan and others in the medical community disagree that genetic research and the resulting drugs will offer a panacea for the most serious medical problems. Callahan (1998, p. 70) writes, "While medical researchers and the for-profit research industry are forever optimistic about the prospect of decisively curing disease, no excitement has quite matched that which genetic research has engendered. The claim in its behalf is sweeping and radical:

genetic research and its clinical application promise to finally bring medicine to the root causes of disease. Once these causal, molecular mechanisms are understood, clinical medicine and medical technology will be in a superb position to eliminate many, if not most, of the deadliest diseases." Callahan adds these words of caution: "The grandiose claims of some of molecular medicine's most ardent proponents must be approached warily: the raising of venture capital requires unrelenting optimism" (p. 71).

We included Callahan's cautionary words because much of what follows definitely has a ring of short-term optimism to it. (There seems to be little disagreement about the long-term potential—2020 and further into the future—for genetics to make major contributions in eliminating many diseases and improving quality of life.) We think that even in the five-year time frame used in this book, there is more to genetic research than Wall Street hype. We believe there is substance behind many of the breakthroughs described in this chapter. Exhibit 9.1 summarizes the key findings of this chapter.

Exhibit 9.1. Highlights in Genetic Research, New Drugs, and Advances in Medical Technology.

- The Human Genome Project, completed ahead of schedule, will lead to advances in genetic testing and new drugs for chronic diseases.

- Personalized medicine—the ability to target treatments and drugs to the needs of the individual—will become common and much more effective than current approaches.

- New drugs will be safer, more powerful, and more selective than ever before. They will also be tremendously expensive.

- Pharmaceutical companies are placing their bets on consumers in terms of demanding new drugs. Pharmaceutical advertising to consumers has increased fourfold since 1994, with no end in sight.

- Even without major technological breakthroughs, we can expect important incremental advancements in medical technology in every medical specialty.

- In terms of driving health care spending, the economic impact of advances in medical technology will be even greater than in the 1990s. This will pose serious issues for health plans, HCFA, and consumers.

Biotechnology

This section focuses on the potential of genetic research to affect the lives of humans through gene therapy and gene-based drugs. Of course, we are also setting the stage for understanding the effects of genetic research, gene therapy, and new drugs on health care providers, consumers, and payers.

Human Genome Project

Congress appropriated funds to begin planning the Human Genome Project in 1988. It was initially anticipated that the endeavor would take fifteen years and cost $3 billion. The project actually began in October 1990. In a lecture to the Massachusetts Medical Society, Francis Collins, M.D., (1999, p. 28) said, "The endeavor was both awesome and chancy. The instruction book— the human genome—was vastly larger than any genetic endowment tackled so far, and in 1990, the tools were not yet powerful enough to perform the task." When the project was launched, its boosters compared it to the Manhattan Project during World War II or "the mission to put men on the moon: an effort so complex and so broad in scope that only the government had the financial and bureaucratic resources to pull it off—yet with such huge potential payoffs that virtually no resources should be spared" (Lemonick and Thompson, 1999, p. 44).

In late 1998 improvements in technology, private sector competition, success in achieving early mapping goals, and a growing demand for the human DNA sequence prompted leaders to move the schedule forward. The result: a working draft by the federal genome team was expected in spring 2000, considerably ahead of schedule.

Four Characteristics of the Project

According to Collins (1999), the Human Genome Project has four characteristics. It must be

- *Accurate.* The DNA spellings must have an accuracy of 99.99 percent or better.

- *Assembled.* The shorter lengths of sequenced DNA must be accurately assembled into longer, genomic-scale pieces that reflect the original genomic DNA.
- *Affordable.* The DNA sequence must be affordable to users; the aim is to reduce cost as much as possible.
- *Accessible.* The high-quality finished DNA sequence should be accessible within twenty-four hours through public databases and the Internet.

On the last point Collins said it is imperative that the results of the project be made available almost instantaneously because "the human DNA sequence arms scientists seeking to understand disease with new information and techniques to unravel the mysteries of human biology" (p. 29). Collins explained, "This knowledge will dramatically accelerate the development of new strategies for the diagnosis, prevention, and treatment of disease, not just for single-gene disorders but for the host of more common complex diseases (e.g., diabetes, heart disease, schizophrenia, and cancer) for which genetic differences may contribute to the risk of contracting the disease and the response to particular therapies" (p. 29).

Competition in Converting Genetic Research into New Drugs

The *Wall Street Journal* reported that former Harvard researcher William Haseltine, chairman and CEO of Human Genome Sciences Inc., shook up the drug industry with a bold vision: that exotic computerized gene-hunting technologies would soon produce an unprecedented cornucopia of new medicines. "Dr. Haseltine's vision contributed to a sea change in the way drug-industry research was conducted, and inspired investors to pour billions of dollars into start-up companies plying similar gene-hunting methods," the article said (Langreth, 1999, p. B1). Referring to the human testing of the first three drugs coming from Haseltine's company, the article went on to say, "The stakes in this endeavor are enormous. Drug manufacturers hope to identify defective or overactive genes that are responsible for numerous major diseases. Based on the gene discoveries, they hope to create new blockbuster medicines that will treat the biochemical causes of disease and trauma, rather than merely alleviating symptoms as most current medications do" (p. B1).

Leland Kaiser, a health care futurist, agrees with the importance of genetic research and its link with new drugs. "This represents one of the most profound technological breakthroughs we have seen this century," Kaiser said. "And it has come faster than many would have expected. I fully expect to see many new drugs capable of treating diseases that couldn't previously be treated. The quality of life of many people will be dramatically improved" (interview, Mar. 31, 1999).

A New Era of "Personalized Medicine"

The *Wall Street Journal* reported on the possibility that a number of large drug companies would jointly fund an effort to supplement the Human Genome Project by focusing on single nucleotide polymorphisms (SNPs), or "snips." Francis Collins, who directs the National Human Genome Project Institute, says, "SNPs serve as a blinking light on DNA sequences showing there is something very interesting here—for example, something that is contributing to diabetes. Finding these SNP variations will thus provide new diagnostic tools and incredibly important clues to new therapies" (Langreth, Waldholz, and Moore, 1999, p. A1). In the same article Allen Roses, vice president and worldwide director of genetic research at Glaxo Wellcome, says, "In the future, before a doctor prescribes a medicine, the doctor will take some blood, have it analyzed at a nearby lab and identify which of, let's say, 12 drugs are most likely to treat the patient effectively with the minimal side effects" (p. A6). Such treatment would not be possible without a computer snip map readily available to doctors.

In a later article the *Wall Street Journal* noted that Glaxo researchers were reported to have identified, or to be close to identifying, three previously unknown genes, using a technology that is rapidly transforming pharmaceutical research. The article stated, "Glaxo hopes that understanding the basic biology behind diabetes, migraines and psoriasis, the vexing skin ailment, will quickly lead it to develop profitable medicines that either treat the illnesses in novel ways, or even help prevent them in genetically vulnerable individuals" (Waldholz and Tanouye, 1999, p. A1).

A *Newsweek* article alluded to the revolutionary customization of drug treatments that genetic research aims to achieve: "License plates are personalized, exercise routines are individualized, even Levi's can be custom cut. . . . Working in the new field called pharmacogenetics, scientists are making discoveries that link particular genes to how patients will respond to medication—specifically, whether the drug will help them and whether they will suffer side effects. The research, says Dr. Michael Kauffman of the biotech firm Millennium Predictive Medicine, promises to 'change the practice of medicine'" (Begley, 1999, p. 66).

Our sense of what consumers want out of the health care system is consistent with these concepts about personalized medicine. Physicians and hospitals will have to respond. However, it will not come cheap.

New Opportunities for Pharmaceutical Companies

The field of genetic research opens up more opportunities for drug companies than they could possibly investigate in the next twenty years. "By the 1990s," *Time* magazine reported, "decades of work had led to the identification of 500 different biological targets for drugs. Thanks to the Human Genome Project, researchers expect to identify another 500 in just the next few years" (Gorman, 1999, p. 80). The key issue for pharmaceutical firms is to prioritize the targets.

Although each pharmaceutical company has its own strategy, there is agreement on three key points:

- Drugs will be safer, more powerful, and much more selective than ever before.
- Physicians will be able to consult a patient's genetic profile to determine ahead of time whether the individual is more likely to respond to one type of medication or another.
- Computers and other digital technologies are going to play a much bigger role in evaluating new research and determining how patients should be treated.

The pharmaceutical giants are eager to exploit the latest genetic information to create new drugs, but they do not see the need to completely reinvent the wheel. The medications they design will still be derived from chemical compounds, or small molecules, that happen to be biologically active. One of the advantages of this approach is that "small molecules won't be destroyed in the stomach, so they can be taken by mouth" (Gorman, 1999, p. 81).

Genetic Testing

Genetic testing is now common. For example, an expectant mother undergoes prenatal screening that involves a sampling of her blood to "seek out telltale proteins that may indicate spina bifida, neural-tube defects or Down syndrome." However, "these tests can spot only visible abnormalities in the 23 pairs of chromosomes we inherit from our parents, such as the extra chromosome associated with Down syndrome" (Golden, 1999a, p. 57).

But thanks to the success of molecular biologists in identifying specific disease genes, genetic centers offer DNA testing for thirty or forty of the more commonly inherited disorders, including cystic fibrosis, Huntington's disease, muscular dystrophy, and various types of degeneration of the brain stem, spinal cord, and peripheral nerves (Golden, 1999a). Wayne Grody, head of the DNA diagnostic lab at the UCLA Medical Center, says, "We'll soon be governed by a new paradigm—genomic medicine—with tests and ultimately treatment for every disease linked to the human genome" (Golden, 1999a, p. 58).

The moral and ethical issues associated with this ability to identify faulty genes and their potential to trigger disease will undoubtedly generate a vigorous debate rivaling abortion and euthanasia. Related to this, there will be serious questions about who pays for these tests, how the test results may be used in providing health insurance coverage, and privacy protection for individuals. The issue of experience rating versus community rating (introduced in Chapter Two) will be part of the continuing policy debate on these issues.

Gene Therapy

Gene therapy is the placement of beneficial genes into the cells of patients. By introducing the gene and the protein it produces, says Inder Verma, a professor at the Salk Institute in La Jolla, California, "you either eliminate the defect, ameliorate the defect, slow down the progression of the disease or in some way interfere with the disease" (Jaroff, 1999, p. 68).

The major limitation of gene therapy is the delivery of the genes to the right cells in the human body. There has been limited success in delivering genes directly into the heart muscle, and many experimental procedures are being tested (Jaroff, 1999, p. 70). Critics of gene therapy point to the slow pace of progress: "These days . . . gene therapy looks unlikely to pay off in a big way anytime soon. . . . From the beginning, the therapy's main difficulty has been a logistical one: how to deliver enough healthy genes to the appropriate site and get them to stay there long enough to cure or alleviate a disease" (Langreth and Moore, 1999, page A1). However, French Anderson of Genetic Therapy Inc. urges patience. "People don't understand that the development of an ordinary drug from time of concept to product is 10 years," he says. "We're talking about a revolutionary approach to therapy, and we're only eight years into it" (Jaroff, 1999a, p. 73).

Stem Cell Research

Medical researchers claim that if the government started funding stem cell research, treatments for diseases such as Parkinson's could be available in as few as five years. "But," as one article points out, "there's a catch; stem cells are generally derived from controversial sources—human embryos. And federal law does not permit federal funds to be spent on this type of research" (Gianelli, 1998, p. 1).

These cells are unique in that they are pluripotent—capable of becoming all the different types of cells and tissue in the body. The goal is that once stem cells are able to be isolated and grown, they can eventually be directed to grow into whatever cells or tissues are desired. Harold Varmus, director of the National Institutes of Health, says, "It is not too unrealistic to say that this research has the potential to revolutionize the practice of medicine and improve the quality and length of life" (Gianelli, 1998, p. 34).

In our judgment the United States will resolve ethical and moral issues and find ways to allow this type of research to continue. Therefore, in looking ahead five years, the results of this research should begin to have significant impact near the end of the period.

Impact of Biotech Research: Summary

One commentator notes a few of the many potential benefits of genetic research: "Gene therapy and gene-based drugs are two ways we could benefit from our growing mastery of genetic science. But there will be others as well, including new kinds of vaccines, new sources of transplant tissue, even techniques doctors may someday use to stave off the aging process" (Lemonick, 1999, p. 89). A key issue of course is how to pay for the potential benefits of genetic research and new drugs. Should the benefits package of health plans be expanded to include these new treatments? Should Medicare cover these new drugs? (This issue is discussed in more detail in Chapter Eleven.)

We believe that part of the answer lies with consumers and their willingness to make trade-offs in selecting various health plan options. If we look at the advertising directed at consumers, apparently the large pharmaceutical companies believe that a substantial number of higher-income individuals will ante up the money needed to purchase the new products being created. But what about individuals and families who cannot afford these new therapies or drugs?

New Drugs and Their Potential Impact

Recent statistics on the sales of new drugs, as well as the bombardment of direct-to-consumer drug advertising in national magazines and on television, have caused a shake-up in the health care industry. For some health plans the cost of drugs now exceeds payments to physicians and may soon be more than the amounts paid to hospitals.

Why the Need for So Many New Drugs?

A report by the Boston Consulting Group (BCG) reveals that "drug products reaching the market today often experience only 50% to 80% average efficacy, and experts estimate that as many as 20% to 50% of prescriptions written today are either ineffective or only marginally effective for the person taking the drug" (Egger, 1999, pp. 1, 22). However, according to the BCG study, the future of health care is tailored drugs for individuals. "Genomics could help eliminate the estimated 20% to 50% of prescriptions that are ineffective—and save more money in overall treatment," the study concludes (p. 22).

How Many New Drugs Can We Expect?

Reports by the BCG and PricewaterhouseCoopers (PWC) indicate that "the pharmaceutical industry will need to produce an increasing number of new products, market them more aggressively, and sell more of them in order to overcome the high cost of research and development and realize even a modest profit in the years ahead" (Egger, 1999, p. 22). The PWC report suggests that the drug companies must launch between twenty-four and thirty-four new drugs over the next seven years, with each one earning $1 billion to $1.45 billion (Egger, 1999).

Will Drugs Reduce Hospital Use?

PWC's Robert McDonald, a former hospital administrator, argues that "many of these drugs in fact reduce costs because they reduce the length of stay and patients get home quicker and they get better quicker." He goes on to say, "So while you may have a more expensive component in pharmaceutical costs, the most expensive part of the system is the hospital stay" (Egger, 1999, p. 22).

McDonald concedes that many in the pharmaceutical industry have not done a very good job of selling the concept that new drugs can actually reduce overall health care costs. McDonald "is convinced that the smart pharmaceutical companies will find ways to build much stronger collaborative relationships with physicians and hospitals to make sure that best practices which incorporate drug therapies to produce best outcomes—and lower overall costs—become a reality" (Egger, 1999, p. 22).

An attorney who works with pharmaceutical companies told us that there is no question that drugs reduce the use of hospitals. "Most people don't like to go to hospitals. They are willing to pay out of their pockets for prescription drugs that prevent a hospitalization."

This attorney's arguments are bolstered by the drop in the share of health care spending on inpatient hospitalization over the past two decades (see Chapter Three).

A Different Perspective on the Cost Impact of New Drugs

The revenues of pharmaceutical companies, however, have been going up rapidly without a corresponding decline in hospital revenues. Over the past few years spending on hospitals and physicians has grown, and drug company revenues have grown even faster—in double digits in terms of percentage increases every year since 1996. Of course, a more relevant question might be, What would have happened to hospital costs absent the development and use of new drugs?

The claim that new drugs will reduce health care spending, specifically the use of hospitals, appears to be unproven. Cost reductions certainly have not been the result with other types of new technology. As noted in Chapter Four, technology continues to be one of the major contributors to growth in overall health care costs, including hospitals.

Direct-to-Consumer Marketing

According to one report drug companies spent $1.3 billion in direct-to-consumer advertising in 1998—a fourfold increase in advertising expenditures since 1994 (Egger, 1999). Some estimates for the year 2000 exceed $2 billion. Leaders of the pharmaceutical industry defend this marketing approach, arguing that it results in better-informed, intelligent consumers and leads to better outcomes. One physician said, "Having better-informed consumers who take more responsibility for their own health has to be beneficial." Others argue that it drives up utilization and causes consumers to request specific brands rather than accepting cheaper generic drugs. (The sale of generic drugs has been flat for a number of years.)

As for who will pay for these new drugs, Leland Kaiser believes that many individuals will buy these new prescription drugs with their own funds. "I don't expect Medicare or private health plans to cover many of these new drugs," Kaiser said. "They are just going to be too expensive" (interview, Mar. 31, 1999).

Advances in Medical Technology

When it comes to new medical technology, most of the advances are likely to fall into these categories (Institute for the Future, 1997):

- *Advances in imaging.* The use of new imaging technologies (such as electron beam CT, harmonic ultrasound, and high-resolution positron emission tomography) to look at the form and function of organs that were once examined only in surgery.
- *Minimally invasive surgery.* The use of miniaturized devices, digitized imaging, and vascular catheters in neurosurgery, cardiology, and interventional radiology.
- *Vaccines.* The use of vaccines to bolster the immune system, target tumors, or immunize against viruses. Delivery methods, including oral and nasal sprays, will simplify the vaccination process.
- *Artificial blood.* The use of recombinant hemoglobin, using *E. coli,* to create a blood substitute.
- *Xenotransplantation.* The transplantation of tissues and organs from animals into humans, primarily in bone marrow and solid organs.

Following are a few brief case studies of a number of technologies that offer new diagnostic and treatment options. These examples are intended to be an overview of the potential for technological advances that are on the horizon.

Beating the Backache

It seems there may be a substitute for the spinal fusion, a procedure endured by about three hundred thousand people each year. According to an article in *Newsweek,* "Early studies suggest that a new treatment called IDET (intradiscal electrothermal annuloplasty) works at least as well as fusion. The difference is that it takes about 15 minutes under local anesthetic. It costs $7,000 instead of $50,000. And patients walk out of the operating suite when it's over" (Cowley, 1999, p. 64).

The secret is an instrument called SpineCath, which consists of a six-inch needle and a fine catheter with a heating element on the end. "After tracing a patient's pain to a particular disc," the article explains, "doctors insert the catheter through the needle and heat it to 194 degrees for 14 to 17 minutes. The heat not only kills the invading nerves but also tightens the surrounding ligaments, creating a new seal" (p. 64). Preliminary results are encouraging: "The technique is still in its infancy—only 700 patients have been treated—but the early results look promising. In small studies, roughly 80 percent of the recipients have enjoyed reduced pain and greater mobility, and half of those taking narcotic painkillers have ended up drug-free" (p. 64). If IDET lives up to its promise after being used on a large number of patients, the financial implications for orthopedic surgeons and some hospitals could be significant.

Stopping Tremors

One of the most significant treatment strategies of the late 1990s was thalamic stimulation, also known as deep brain stimulation, for patients with Parkinson's disease or essential tremor. The neuronal circuits responsible for tremors are located in the thalamus, a part of the brain. Once this area has been located in a patient, a stimulating electrode is put in place and an extension lead is tunneled under the scalp down to an impulse generator implanted under the skin, just like a heart pacemaker (O'Brien, 1998–1999, p. 5). The results are dramatic. When the patient activates the stimulator, the shaking stops immediately. Patients who could not hold a cup of coffee without spilling it are perfectly calm.

In discussing this procedure and the related equipment, Christopher O'Brien, medical director of the Colorado Neurological Institute's Movement Disorders Center, told us that it costs about $30,000 to perform the tests and surgery and to purchase the equipment. He noted that Medicare and most health plans will pay for deep brain stimulation. Previously, many patients had paid for the procedure out of their pockets. "Research into stimulation of other regions of the brain," O'Brien said, "is leading to many promising new applications; however, we expect continuing issues relating to who pays. The technology is moving faster than Medicare and health plans' ability to consider coverage, and this will lead to consumers having to consider paying for these technologies."

Healing Heart Disease

On the same day two different newspaper articles covered approaches to dealing with heart disease. One related to blocking the flow of blood to tumors, and the other concerned plaque in the blood vessels leading to the heart. These two articles are representative of what we can expect to read, almost on a daily basis, over the next five years. The implications of these examples for women, obstetrician gynecologists, heart surgeons, and hospitals are profound.

Fibroids

Fibroids are benign tumors typically occurring in the uterus. More than two hundred thousand women in the United States have hysterectomies each year because of fibroids, so it is a significant problem and one that requires large use of health care resources. Fibroid embolization, a new technique, shrinks the fibroids by blocking their blood supply. Although the procedure is in its early stages of development and is controversial, Gaylene Pron of the University of Toronto, coordinator of a center on fibroid embolization, says, "Women want this, or, rather, they don't want surgery. This is a women-driven technology" (Gilbert, 1999, p. A12). This is another example of the power of the consumer in action.

Artery-Clogging Deposits

In his laboratory at Children's Hospital in Boston, Judah Folkman has performed experiments that block the blood supply to plaque in the arteries. "The finding that turning off blood-vessel growth keeps the plaque from growing—that's a big, important step in understanding the science that could lead to new treatment," Folkman says (Winslow, 1999b, p. B1). He also acknowledges that more research is needed before the connection between blood vessel formation and heart diseases in humans can be established.

Economic Impact of Medical Technology

Almost everyone who has attempted to assess the reasons for the increase in health care spending in the United States has concluded that the steady growth of new technology and its application are probably the most important factors. (See Chapter Four.)

Incremental Change

William Schwartz, professor of medicine at the University of Southern California and a well-known author and speaker on the subject of medical technology, says that there have been medical advances that represent quantitative leaps in medical science.

"Even the least knowledgeable patient," Schwartz (1998, p. 22) says, "has probably heard about ultrasound and bypass surgery. By contrast, the thousands of small improvements that have collectively transformed medical specialties like anesthesia or neonatal intensive care receive relatively little public attention." Schwartz describes the development of technology in these and other fields, amply illustrating the point that incremental growth of technology in health care has been truly impressive. He expects many incremental—and important—advances in the future.

Diffusion of Medical Technology

Victor Fuchs, a highly regarded health care economist, studied the diffusion of seven frequently used medical procedures in 1987 and 1995 and the rates of change between those years. The procedures were angioplasty, coronary artery bypass graft, cardiac catheterization, carotid endarterectomy, hip replacement, knee replacement, and laminectomy. "All seven procedures," he reported, "showed substantial increases in utilization between 1987 and 1995 for both sexes at all ages. Even the rapid diffusion of angioplasty, which was expected to obviate the need for coronary artery bypass graft (CABG) for many patients, did not result in lower utilization of the latter procedure" (Fuchs, 1999, pp. 13–14).

Fuchs noted that none of the seven procedures was a breakthrough in 1987. "Instead, as physicians developed greater confidence and capacity to perform the procedures on more patients, especially on older patients, utilization steadily increased" (p. 13). He also observed that most of the growth in use of technology in health care probably follows this pattern.

Economic Consequences: Conclusions

What began as high-tech procedures only offered in tertiary care centers in larger metropolitan areas have become commonplace in regional medical centers and community hospitals. We have observed this pattern over and over—in cardiac catheterization, angioplasty, and coronary artery bypass grafts, for example.

In our view the growth of medical technology is accelerating and will continue to accelerate rapidly in the early part of the new millennium. Consumers will demand it and want the benefits. All of this will drive up health care spending, and consumers will be faced with the need to pay for access to the technology. We do not believe that any system of rationing access to demonstrably beneficial technology will be acceptable in the United States.

Who will make the decisions on what consumers will have access to and what will be restricted? In countries with national health care systems, it would be a public policy decision. In the United States we believe that these kinds of decisions will increasingly be made by consumers, based on the kinds of health plans they purchase and what they are willing to pay for out of their pockets.

What About Basic Health Care?

With all the attention focused on the Internet, new medical technology, genetic research, targeted drugs, and advanced health care information technology, are we forgetting about old-fashioned, basic health care and prevention? This is a growing concern, particularly in a country that has many people with unhealthy habits, has large numbers of seniors who do not receive adequate preventive care, and accepts the fact that forty-five million people are uninsured.

Preventive Care for the Elderly

"Elderly Need Preventive Care, but Don't Get It" was the headline of a *Wall Street Journal* article identifying many deficiencies in basic health care services for the elderly. The article focused on the results of the third edition of *The Dartmouth Atlas of Health Care*, a compendium that tracks, by geographical area, how health care services are provided.

Dr. John Wennberg, lead author of the *Dartmouth Atlas*, said the findings "suggest that better management and not more spending is the crucial missing ingredient in the delivery of preventive care for the elderly." He added, "There are no systems in place for doctors to take care of patient populations. Primary care is chaotically organized and so is hospital care" (Winslow, 1999a, p. B4). Wennberg also noted, "These are cheap services and the benefits are obvious. There is no system of quality in place to insure that these simple things get done" (p. B1).

Good Health Practices

Daniel Callahan, whom we quoted at the beginning of this chapter, expresses concern about the disparity between an informed populace and poor basic health habits:

> I find it one of the great puzzles these days that we're getting much more sophisticated lay people. They know how to use the Web, usually to get information about medical technology and drugs. But meanwhile the prevention statistics look horrible—exercise is down, obesity is up, smoking is not going away. Somehow, we don't seem to have gotten anywhere with the most primitive stuff, whereas everybody's going to get smart as hell about looking up the likely side-effects of their hypertension medicine, having lived a lousy life prior to getting the hypertension. How do you change this behavior? ["The Future of Health Care," 1999, p. 49].

Basic Medical Services Are the Most Important

Arthur Jones, a surgeon practicing at Exempla Lutheran Medical Center in Wheat Ridge, Colorado, told us, "A lot of what you have been describing in terms of technological advances and consumerism is true, but it is on the periphery of medicine. Most of what we do is the nuts and bolts of caring for people. Regardless of how much use people make of the Internet, or how genetic research affects new drugs, the vast majority of patients will still have the same old medical problems. It is our business to focus on treating these illnesses" (interview, Apr. 13, 1999).

We do not disagree with this assessment or with Callahan's. However, based on what we have discussed thus far in this book, we conclude that basic health care is likely to be enhanced through the use of the Internet, drug company advertising, clinical information systems (which could, for example, generate reminders that elderly patients are due for certain tests or screenings), disease management programs, and other technological advances. Much information will be available for people who want to help themselves, something that will be more appreciated as the United States moves steadily toward a consumer-dominated and consumer-financed health care system.

Self-Help and Encouragement

Andrew Grove, the founder of Intel, suggests that Americans will get much more of their basic health care information over the Internet and that their support systems will come from the same source (see Chapter Six). The Institute for the Future (1999, p. 2) comes to a similar conclusion: "Think of the Web of the future as an English pub. The English go there to drink, but they could buy beer at any liquor store and drink it in the comfort of their own homes. So the most successful pubs create an atmosphere and a community that invites 'regulars' to return. . . . Health plans and providers will have to work in the same direction if they are going to use cyberspace successfully." Leland Kaiser told us he sees the role of physicians as encouragers, counselors, and facilitators of this process. All this adds up to more personal responsibility for basic health care.

Disease Management

We have been impressed with the efforts of several disease management programs to educate and encourage patients and to monitor the progress of the patients they work with, most of whom have chronic diseases. Disease management strikes us as a fairly basic—and badly needed—service aimed at helping those with chronic diseases deal with the day-to-day problems of eating right, taking medication, exercising, and taking other actions that will improve their quality of life.

Telehealth and Remote Care

As discussed in Chapter Eight, the potential for telehealth is enormous, especially for older Americans and those suffering with chronic diseases. It seems to us that telehealth could work in conjunction with home health and disease management programs.

We realize of course that loneliness and boredom are part of the reason older Americans like to meet with their physicians. It gives them the incentive to get dressed and leave the house and provides someone with whom they can discuss their aches and pains. Telehealth will have to find a substitute for this type of interpersonal experience, and perhaps the answer lies in the chat rooms and support groups accessible on the Internet. Our experience indicates that older Americans will increasingly use the Internet and e-mail; this technology will not be limited to younger persons.

Basic Health Care Implications: Summary

In our view many of the advanced communications systems, new drugs, and clinical information systems are likely to have their greatest impact on the more basic types of health care services. Something as simple yet critically important as monitoring the drugs taken by patients, especially seniors, will be extremely valuable in avoiding overdoses and the related problem of taking multiple and potentially interacting medications. Home health, one of the most basic services in health care, could be radically changed—and improved—by telehealth and remote sensing. Simple reminder systems (for such things as mammograms or colectoral cancer screening) for use by physicians who care for an elderly population would be tremendously helpful.

Conclusions

It is impossible to fully anticipate the impact of genetic research, new drugs, and advances in medical technology. In writing this book we picked up new articles and studies dealing with these types of changes on literally a daily basis, many in the *Wall Street Journal,* national newsmagazines, and local newspapers.

There are those who are skeptical about the significance of some of what we have described in this chapter. Daniel Callahan (1998, p. 72) writes, "Genetics and molecular medicine have made remarkable progress to date, but they have a long way to go before they come anywhere near the claims made in their behalf. . . . The genetic revolution is still an idea—an interesting and important idea, but not yet far enough along for us to declare that it has found even in theory the answer to death, sickness, and aging." Despite Callahan's warnings (and we do not take them lightly), it is our view that what is developing today is a reliable and useful indicator of what the future holds—a steady stream of new innovations offering Americans and many people around the world the promise of relief from chronic diseases, higher quality of life, and increased longevity.

We believe the major issues will be the cost of new drugs and medical procedures and the way patients will pay for them. These will be among the most important policy issues of the next decade or more. It is also obvious that new drugs and advances in medical technology will have profound impact on the number of patients in hospitals. Even with the aging of the population, the need for inpatient beds is likely to continue to decline. Despite reports of short-term shortages of hospital beds in California, Minnesota, and other areas, there is nothing we see on the horizon that would counter this long-term downward trend.

The kinds of changes we can reasonably anticipate in health care consolidation are also likely to have profound impact on health care in the twenty-first century. In Chapter Ten we discuss issues revolving around the consolidation, structure, and ownership of medical groups, hospitals, and health plans.

Trends in Consolidation, Ownership, and Capacity

*Currently, there are many areas of healthcare where
competition will remove capacity and produce
consolidation. These changes will be resisted because
of the pain and vested interests of many constituencies.*
JOHN KOSTER, CEO, PROVIDENCE HEALTH SYSTEM,
WASHINGTON, March 1999

Among the external factors affecting health care in the future, the
consolidation of hospitals, physicians, medical groups, and health
plans ranks high in importance. A related issue is ownership: investor
owned versus not-for-profit. When we talk about consolidation trends,
it is also important to assess supply and demand for hospital and
physician services. It has been widely recognized for years that hospitals have too many beds, and some find it puzzling that the capacity of hospitals has not declined more rapidly. Among physicians
there is a surplus of both primary care doctors and specialists, and
in some metropolitan areas a glut of specialists is especially troublesome. This chapter assesses consolidation, ownership, and capacity
as three interrelated external factors affecting local health care markets in the new millennium. Exhibit 10.1 summarizes trends in hospital, medical group, and health plan consolidation.

Hospital Consolidation

The almost continuous consolidation in the health care marketplace represents one of the most dominant trends of the past two

decades. The number of hospital mergers and acquisitions increased from 92 in 1994 to 144 in 1998. The highest number of hospital deals—197—occurred in 1997. About three-fourths of the consolidations were among not-for-profit hospitals and multihospital systems (Cochrane, 1999a).

Sandy Lutz and E. Preston Gee (1998) describe health care industry consolidation in their book *Columbia/HCA: Healthcare on Overdrive.* "With hospitals and physicians falling in line on a grand scale," they write, "[Richard] Scott was playing a tune that Wall Street loved. The lyrics read, 'rapid consolidation of a large and

Exhibit 10.1. Highlights in Hospital, Medical Group, and Health Plan Consolidation.

- Hospital consolidation rates were high in the mid-1990s and have since slowed down. It is unlikely that future consolidation rates will match those of the earlier peak period.

- The results of hospital consolidation have been disappointing in many cases, primarily because of cultural difficulties and an inability to achieve economies of scale.

- Driven by PPMs, hospital acquisition of primary care practices, and a desire to gain market clout with payers, physician and medical group consolidation have been strong over the past decade. Despite the well-publicized problems of PPMs and hospital-affiliated practices, we expect physician consolidation to continue.

- Health plan consolidation appears to be leading to the development of a limited number of very large plans and to the presence of two to four dominant plans in each major market.

- The role of Wall Street capital in the consolidation of hospitals and medical groups has led to mixed results and to some destabilization of health care in local markets.

- Physician supply and demand varies by region, with some metropolitan areas reporting twice as many medical specialists as needed while rural areas have continuing shortages of physicians. Overall, however, there is a growing surplus of physicians.

- In the new millennium it appears that the structure of all aspects of healthcare will move in the direction of larger organizations. This will be driven by market and competitive pressures, the cost of IT, and consumer demands for a greater variety of services.

fragmented market.' In healthcare, that consolidation was happening in a variety of niches: home healthcare, surgery centers, physician groups, and ambulance services. But no other niche carried the clout, the dollars, and the potential for profits as the hospital industry" (p. 82).

In the early 1980s we heard about the potential development of the "supermeds," four large investor-owned (then called "proprietary") chains: Hospital Corporation of America (HCA), American Medical International (AMI), Humana, and National Medical Enterprises. By the early 1990s, for a variety of reasons, most of these organizations were out of the picture or entirely reorganized.

Following is a case study of how a combination of consolidation and shifting fortunes of investor-owned and not-for-profit ownership has affected a major health care system in Colorado.

Presbyterian/St. Luke's Hospital

In Denver, Presbyterian (a not-for-profit hospital) merged with St. Luke's (another not-for-profit) in the early 1980s to form a three-hospital system that included Presbyterian/St. Luke's, with 463 beds, and the 146-bed Presbyterian Medical Center in Aurora, an eastern suburb. In 1985 AMI made the Presbyterian/St. Luke's board an offer it could not refuse—$178 million that would be used to create a foundation called The Colorado Trust. Assets of The Colorado Trust were $350 million as of the end of 1999, making it the second largest charitable foundation in the state.

AMI Runs into Trouble

By 1989, however, AMI began to run into financial difficulties. In fact, AMI was in the midst of building a new $200 million "hospital of the future" on the Presbyterian/St. Luke's downtown campus when construction suddenly stopped. For several days the mystery of the half-completed hospital dominated local news, but then the facts emerged: AMI did not have the financing to complete the project and was in negotiations with the original Presbyterian/St. Luke's board for them to repurchase the hospital by assuming its debts and completing the construction of the new building.

In 1990 the new board had successfully arranged debt financing to accept the AMI offer, and Presbyterian/St. Luke's was once again in the fold of not-for-profit community hospitals, albeit with substantially more debt than five years earlier. However, the community appeared to benefit. The hospital was returned to local ownership, thus retaining an estimated $20 million a year that had been leaving the state for AMI's coffers. The Colorado Trust was supporting numerous social and health care initiatives that benefited residents of Colorado. And construction on the downtown hospital resumed, to be completed in 1991.

Presbyterian/St. Luke's and Swedish Join to Form HealthOne

Three years later, in 1993, the boards and management of Presbyterian/St. Luke's and Swedish Medical Center, a 328-bed not-for-profit located in the southern part of the Denver metropolitan area, announced that they would be merging to create HealthOne, the largest hospital system in Colorado. Many local health care observers considered this a way for the board of Presbyterian/ St. Luke's to spread its inordinate debt over a larger base of assets and revenues.

HealthOne and Columbia Form a Partnership

Within two years, in 1995, HealthOne entered into a partnership arrangement with Columbia/HCA, which owned three other hospitals in the Denver area. The HealthOne board members were quick to point out that this was not a sale but a 50-50 partnership. However, within months, the signs on the hospitals began to change. Swedish Medical Center, a VHA Inc. shareholder and fierce defender of the benefits of community-owned not-for-profit hospitals, became Columbia Swedish Medical Center. In this process the people of the Denver area received the benefits of a small foundation (with about $10 million in assets) but nothing compared to the $178 million associated with the 1985 sale to AMI. But this was not the end of the story.

Columbia/HCA Backs Off

In 1998 it was announced that the Columbia signs were coming down and that Presbyterian/St. Luke's and Swedish Medical Center would be using their former names. How will the story end? In 1999 it was reported that this system had just refinanced $485 million in debt. It would not surprise most people in the Denver area if Swedish and Presbyterian/St. Luke's again reverted to community not-for-profit hospital status.

Is this sort of change good for the employees of these organizations and the physicians who practice at these hospitals? Will the ownership patterns of these hospitals continue this roller-coaster course? Many of the physicians and employees do not like the changes and see no benefits to them or to patients.

Columbia/HCA Nationally

Richard Scott and Richard Rainwater founded Columbia in 1987, and this organization reached its zenith ten years later, when Columbia/HCA was the seventh largest employer in the United States and a favorite of Wall Street. A review of the table of contents of any issue of *Modern Healthcare* from 1995 through 1998 provides evidence of the dominance of Columbia/HCA.

But in mid-1997 the roof fell in as a result of a federal investigation of alleged overbilling and other fraudulent practices by executives and managers of some Columbia/HCA facilities. Under pressure from the board Richard Scott and David Vandewater, chief operating officer, resigned (Lutz and Gee, 1998). As the 1990s closed, Columbia/HCA had ceased acquiring and building hospitals and had begun divesting itself of a number of its properties.

Other Indications of Problems in Hospital Consolidation

Here is the way the *Wall Street Journal* reported on hospital consolidation: "Just a few years ago, mergers were touted as a panacea for troubled hospitals. Combine a couple of major nonprofit facilities, the thinking went, and the result would be an institution capable of withstanding cutthroat competition, pressure from managed care and anticipated Medicare cuts. It hasn't worked out that way" (Lagnado, 1999, p. B7). The article goes on to describe a number of troubled mergers, including Beth Israel and Deaconess in Boston, Columbia Presbyterian Medical and New York Hospital, and hospitals affiliated with Stanford University and the University of California in San Francisco.

Many of the roadblocks to mergers relate to the difficulties of realizing economies of scale. To keep the peace, executives of merged organizations often fail to make tough decisions on eliminating or combining jobs. Additional layers of corporate overhead add to expenses. Furthermore, the drain on resources from integrating information systems, business processes, and clinical programs often places organizations on hold for months. As a result, focus on the market and cost-effectiveness often gets lost. This is borne out by research showing that many merged hospitals fail to realize the financial savings projected prior to the consolidation.

Continuing Hospital Consolidation

By the end of the 1990s there were 6,000 acute care hospitals in the United States. Of these, 1,800 were part of VHA Inc., an alliance of not-for-profit hospitals, and another 1,700 were in Premier, an alliance dominated by not-for-profit multihospital systems. Both of these alliances had experienced substantial growth in the 1980s.

Several of the largest not-for-profit multihospital systems included Ascension Health (73 facilities), Catholic Health Initiatives (70 facilities), Lutheran Health Systems (66 facilities), Sutter (22 facilities), Intermountain Health Care (18 facilities), Sisters of Providence on the West Coast and Alaska (17 facilities), Allina in the Twin Cities (12 facilities), and Advocate in Chicago (8 facilities) (American Hospital Association, 1998; Bellandi, 1999). Columbia/HCA, the largest of the investor-owned hospital systems, had 320 facilities. Other for-profit hospital systems included Tenet (120 facilities), Quorum (22 owned facilities and 237 managed facilities), HealthSouth (73 facilities), Vencor (33 facilities), and Paracelsus (22 facilities) (American Hospital Association, 1998).

Where Is Hospital Consolidation Headed?

Has hospital consolidation run its course, or is there room for additional consolidation over the next five years? Jeffrey Barbakow, chairman and CEO of Tenet, believes that the boom in hospital consolidation is over. "Fast forward with me, for a moment, to the not-too-distant future," Barbakow proposes. "Consolidation—that rallying cry during the 1980s and 1990s for so many major U.S. industries seeking to improve their global competitiveness—has gone about as far as it is going. For the hospital industry, this means that most inefficiencies have been squeezed out of what was once a highly fragmented, wasteful system. Purchasing leverage has been maximized. Administrative efficiencies have been captured. Capacity has been carefully rationalized" (Gilkey, 1999, pp. 93–94).

Barbakow believes that this future has just about arrived. He notes that the American Hospital Association found that about half of all member hospitals consider themselves to be part of a system, compared with 11 percent in 1993. Therefore, Barbakow asserts, the real question is, What comes after consolidation (Gilkey, 1999)?

Our experience indicates that although hospital consolidation has slowed, it will continue. Despite the need for many organizations to become market leaders or improve their competitive positions, the rate of hospital consolidation in the future is unlikely to match that of the last five years. We agree with Barbakow that many of the inefficiencies of hospitals have been squeezed out. What remains is inappropriate utilization and too many hospitals.

Physician and Medical Group Consolidation

The consolidation taking place among physicians and medical groups over the past two decades has not received the press coverage of hospital consolidation, but it has been every bit as important. The same arguments used to justify hospital consolidation were used for physicians and small medical groups—the need to bring together a highly fragmented cottage industry, enhance market clout, improve cost-effectiveness, and generate or attract capital.

The number of medical groups with one hundred or more physicians increased from 189 in 1991 to an estimated 218 by 1997. Many health care industry experts continue to assert that the days of the solo practitioner are gone. Figure 10.1 shows the consolidation of medical groups from 1991 through 1997.

Although we do not have data specifically relating to hospital ownership of medical groups, the acquisition of primary care and multispecialty groups by hospitals during the 1990s contributed to this consolidation. Also, as discussed later in this chapter, the

**Figure 10.1. Growth in the Number of
Larger Medical Groups, 1990–1997.**

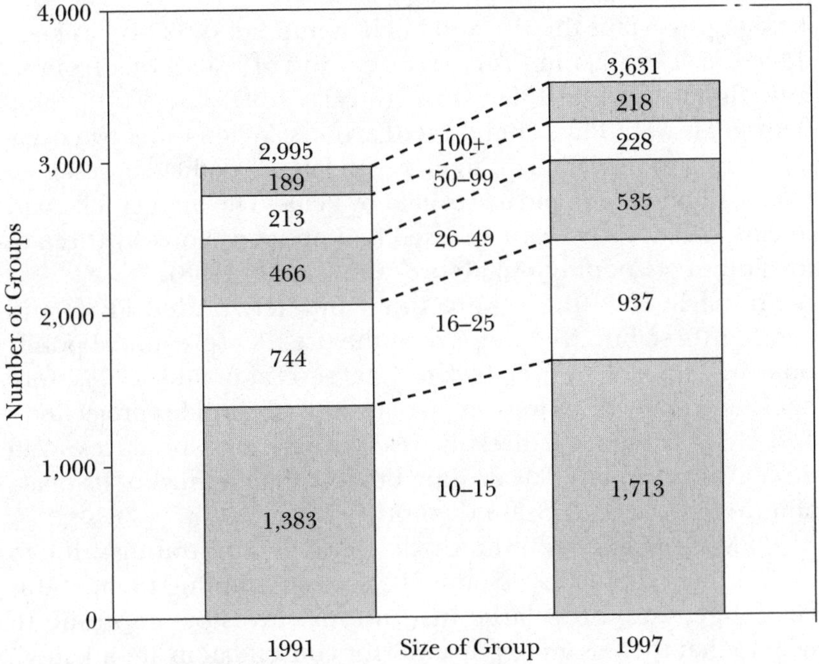

Sources: American Medical Association, 1993; 1999a, p. 10.

growth of PPMs during the past decade added to physician consolidation.

Managed Care Has Been Driving Physician Consolidation

It is generally agreed that managed care has been the driving force in physician and medical group consolidation. There has been an effort on the part of groups of physicians to develop "market clout" in order to deal with health plans. There continues to be a fear that major health plans will not contract with a single physician or small groups and a belief that therefore physicians need to consolidate their practices or join IPAs, PHOs, management services organizations (MSOs), or take some other organized approach to the delivery and financing of medicine.

Physician Practice Management Companies Were the Primary Consolidators

Among physicians the rise and fall of a number of PPMs has been dramatic. The PPM industry was a darling of Wall Street from its founding in the mid-1980s through early 1997. The most prominent PPMs were PhyCor and MedPartners. When these two organizations announced plans to merge in late 1997, they represented half of all physicians and assets held by PPMs. The merger fell apart in early 1998. PPMs were assessed in a previous book by three of the authors (Coddington, Moore, and Clarke, 1998).

In early 1998 there were thirty publicly traded PPMs and another three hundred or more in the pre-IPO (pre–initial public offering) stage. However, by late 1999 several notable PPMs were bankrupt, many PPMs were falling far short of earnings projections, and MedPartners was divesting itself of physician practices. Wall Street valuation of PPMs dropped to less than a third of its peak, and there were no IPOs on the horizon.

PPMs are faced with the challenge of demonstrating value to their affiliated practices. Some PPMs are attempting to meet this challenge, and a few large institutional investors continue to believe that there is an opportunity for consolidation among medical groups.

Unionization of Physicians

Is the movement among physicians to unionize, embraced in mid-1999 by the American Medical Association (AMA), another aspect of the consolidation of physicians? We think it is. Unionization is a way of gaining clout with managed care plans, hospitals, and any other entity that threatens the autonomy and incomes of physicians.

At the same time we need to realize that only a fraction of all physicians are eligible to join unions. A physician-leader of a large organization told us, "This only applies to employed physicians. Those in professional corporations would not be eligible to join a union. Employed physicians represent about one-seventh of all physicians."

Physician Consolidation: Summary

Despite the slowdown in PPM and hospital acquisitions of physician practices, we anticipate continuing consolidation among physicians and medical groups. In many respects the PPMs sensed a need for physician practices to consolidate in order to gain access to capital, improve their operating efficiencies, and acquire greater bargaining power with managed care plans. In other words consolidation pressures for physicians and medical groups are real and unlikely to disappear anytime soon.

Health Plan Consolidation

In summarizing the trend toward health plan and provider consolidation, Uwe Reinhardt, economics professor at Princeton and a well-known health care speaker, made this observation: "The health system is stumbling toward a bilateral monopoly of insurance companies and provider groups in every market. If only one insurer is left to deal with local doctors and hospitals, they will send the bill to the consumer by raising premiums" (Cochrane, 1998, p. 1).

Mergers and Acquisitions

In support of Reinhardt's point there were ninety-four mergers and acquisitions among health plans between 1993 and 1998. These included FHP's acquisition of TakeCare, PacifiCare's acquisition of FHP, and Aetna's purchase of three health plans: U.S. Healthcare, Prudential HealthCare, and NYLife Care. United HealthCare, Aetna, and CIGNA have the capital to make additional acquisitions (Kalamas, Pinkus, Wang, and Zino, 1999).

Anthem Moves East and West

Anthem, a mutually owned plan based in Indianapolis, is one of the most aggressive BCBS systems. In 1999 Anthem insured five million people in a variety of traditional and managed care plans in Ohio, Kentucky, Connecticut, and New York. It was attempting to acquire plans in Maine, New Hampshire, and Rhode Island.

According to a spokesperson for Anthem, the company has to stay big to compete in the health plan game: "Three years ago we thought $5 billion was big enough. Now we probably have to be a $10 billion company" (Gentry, 1999a). As part of its western strategy, Anthem acquired BCBS of Colorado. This system was one of the top four health plans in Colorado, with over four hundred thousand covered lives. (This compares with almost one million customers in the early 1980s, before the advent of managed care.)

Although additional health plan consolidation will occur, primarily absorbing smaller plans on a market-by-market basis, it appears to us that on a national scale opportunities for consolidation may be diminishing. (Future health plan consolidation is part of the scenarios considered in Chapter Thirteen.)

Investor-Owned Hospitals, Medical Groups, and Health Plans

The recent track record of large investor-owned hospital systems, such as Columbia/HCA and Quorum, has caused some health care policymakers and investment analysts to lose confidence in this ownership and financing approach for hospitals and medical groups. Investor-owned consolidated groups must prove that they can bring sufficient value added to justify the capital invested.

A big part of the problem is meeting Wall Street expectations for ever-increasing revenues and earnings. This of course is the basis for establishing the price-earnings multiple for most stocks. We have already seen the troubles experienced by Columbia/HCA and many publicly owned PPMs when they failed to meet investors' expectations.

For most health plans, hospitals, and medical groups, there are numerous external variables that make it extremely difficult to produce increased revenues and earnings year in and year out. For health plans there is the historical underwriting cycle of three good years followed by three poor ones (see Chapter Three). Hospitals that push hard to increase earnings by cutting costs run the risk of angering employees, physicians, and patients. For most medical groups outside pressures on billing rates, and the coming and going of physicians, make predictability difficult. And Wall Street tends to set high financial expectations.

Community Not-for-Profit Hospitals Can Usually Adjust

In the present health care payment system most community not-for-profit hospitals or multihospital systems are at financial risk for their performance. They do not have a partner with deep pockets and generally can only raise capital through internal funds or debt. If they have several consecutive good years, they accumulate cash reserves that can be used for new technology, renovation of older facilities, and expansion. When the inevitable poor years hit, they reduce operating expenses or draw on reserves. But this is a community decision reflected by the hospital board. Community boards tend to set lower financial expectations. In addition, some community hospitals in rural areas have been able to fall back on taxpayer support. Without this type of support, many small hospitals will not be able to survive in the future.

Medical Groups Are Flexible

Physicians in most medical groups are also responsible for their own financial performance. If earnings are down, bonuses and other cash distributions usually go by the board; there may even be salary cuts and layoffs. In good times physicians can increase their take-home pay or set aside reserves (this rarely happens, but we see a tiny trend developing).

Health Plans

Some of the largest health plans are part of much larger insurance companies, like Aetna U.S. Healthcare and CIGNA, and are able to weather the wide fluctuations in earnings inherent in health insurance. The more focused health plans have incentives to merge with stronger plans, to improve market positioning, gain more leverage over providers, and increase financial reserves. These types of organizations need access to outside equity capital. However, shareholders should expect wild rides in terms of share price fluctuations.

Oxford Health Plan Debacle

The pattern of a Wall Street love affair and divorce can be seen in the story of the Oxford Health Plan:

[Oxford] pursued market share by offering patients generous benefits and paying most affiliated doctors on a fee-for-service basis—a relatively light-handed form of managed care. The company advertised aggressively, targeting a relatively young, affluent population in the hope that favorable selection would offset the liberal benefits and payments to physicians. The company grew from under 100,000 subscribers in 1992 to 2 million subscribers in late 1996. . . . For a time, Oxford was the darling of Wall Street. Its chief executive officer, Stephen Wiggins, was an apostle of shareholder-owned HMOs who regularly denounced nonprofit plans as inefficient tax evaders. Wiggins's formula seemed too good to be true, and it was. . . . By the third quarter of 1997, the company was reporting a medical loss ratio of nearly 100 percent and had to delay its payments to doctors. The problem was blamed on computer foul-ups, but in part it reflected overly sanguine business strategy [Kuttner, 1998a, pp. 1561–1562].

For-Profit Versus Not-for-Profit: Summary

For hospitals and medical groups, evidence supporting the investor-owned model appears to ebb and flow with the fortunes of industry leaders. If the leaders are strong and growing, the experts predict a movement toward this ownership model. In bad times, however, these same experts are likely to believe that all investor-owned companies will go bust. The truth is somewhere in the middle: given proper leadership, either investor-owned or nonprofit hospitals and medical groups can prosper in the changing health care scene.

This brief analysis of investor ownership is not intended to cover other types of health care organizations—drug companies, Internet start-ups, long-term care, vision and dental care, rehabilitation, and other medical services. We have focused on investor ownership of medical groups and hospitals, which we characterize as unimpressive, and health plans, where it makes more sense.

Hospital Beds: Supply and Demand

Our research indicates that there are a number of networking, or collaborative, relationships among competing hospitals around the country. In some cases these kinds of efforts have met with antitrust concerns, but in general they appear to be in the interests of the community.

The Experience of One Community

One of the authors worked with the board of directors of the smaller hospital in a two-hospital town with a population of one hundred thousand. Although good arguments could be made for savings from the hospitals' being under single ownership, the board believed that the people in the community wanted a choice.

The two hospitals were known for their collaboration. The CEO of the smaller hospital said, "I believe that many of the potential cost savings of merging have already been achieved simply by the two of us working together. We do different things and don't compete on very many services. We jointly own the home health service and we continue to evaluate other opportunities for working together."

Excess Hospital Capacity: Is It a Problem?

Our conclusion is that the excess capacity of acute care hospitals is not a significant problem in terms of driving up costs or lowering quality. This is not to say that there are not opportunities for hospitals to combine or to find ways to collaborate for the benefit of the community.

Physicians: Supply and Demand

The perceived surplus of medical specialists, which is especially acute in some metropolitan areas, is an important factor influencing the health care environment of the future. But what is the overall situation with respect to physician supply and demand?

An Argument That Physicians Are Not in Oversupply

Nelson Tilden, senior executive director of Medical Search Institute/Superior Consultants, argues that there is no physician surplus and that one is unlikely to develop. "I contend," says Tilden, "that we absolutely do not have an oversupply of physicians in this country. Not only don't we have a glut, we will have a short-age in 10 years" (Moore, 1999, p. 3).

As evidence to support his viewpoint, Tilden points to the low number of physicians actually working full time. He says that less than 25 percent of all doctors are full-time equivalents (FTEs) but that most are counted as FTEs in surveys. He adds that growing numbers of female physicians account for a portion of the trend toward part-time work. Other physicians are working shorter hours because they are partially retired, disabled, or have different priorities. Tilden also believes that many physicians will soon leave the profession (Moore, 1999).

A More Traditional View of the "Physician Glut"

Thomas Bodenheimer believes that evidence of an oversupply of physicians, particularly specialists, is strong. Of the six hundred thousand physicians engaged in patient care in 1996, 70 percent were specialists. "By the year 2000," Bodenheimer (1999, p. 587) said, "the number of physicians caring for patients will have increased to 203 per 100,000 population, as compared with 115 per 100,000 in 1970. This growth in the physician-to-population ratio is attributable to increased numbers of specialists."

Bodenheimer noted that a 1994 study found that only 112 physicians per hundred thousand of population would be needed as of the year 2000, leading to a surplus of 165,000 physicians. "A more commonly accepted estimate," Bodenheimer explained, "is that given by the Council on Graduate Medical Education, which proposed that 60 to 80 generalists and 85 to 105 specialists (a total of 145 to 185 physicians) per 100,000 population would be needed by 2000" (p. 587). He also went on to note that the supply of physician's assistants and advance-practice nurses is expected to number 168,000 in the year 2005.

Physician Supply and Demand Is a Regional Issue

There are tremendous regional variations in the supply and demand of physicians. For example, Missoula, Montana, has eighteen orthopedic surgeons for a metro area of about 100,000 residents and a service area representing an additional 150,000; by most measures this is about twice as many as needed. Other rural areas lack adequate orthopedic coverage.

Some areas that have had significant surplus of physicians now find themselves in balance. For example, the Portland, Oregon, metropolitan area, which has traditionally had an oversupply of physicians, has seen the pendulum swing in the other direction. Greg Van Pelt of Providence Health System attributes the outflow of physicians to "issues relating to managed care, the declining fortunes of some PPMs, and better economic opportunities elsewhere. In a sense we have had a 'brain drain'" (interview, Aug. 10, 1999).

The situation in the Los Angeles area is just the opposite. An internal medicine physician in Pasadena, head of a large IPA, told us that there were twice as many cardiologists and members of his organization in his area as needed. "Of course," this physician said, "when we decided to capitate cardiologists, this made it a lot easier to get them to go along with it."

Many rural areas continue to be short of physicians. Bodenheimer (1999) noted that rural areas—with 20 percent of the U.S. population—have only 9 percent of the nation's physicians. "Inner cities are similarly underserved," he said (p. 587).

Primary Care: Is There a Shortage?

A 1993 article in the *New England Journal of Medicine* portrayed the conventional thinking at the time of the Clinton health care reform debate: "The United States is in the process of rediscovering primary care. Primary care is being promoted as an antidote to excessive health care costs and inadequate access to health services. However, primary care physicians in the United States are perceived to be in short supply, and their number is dwindling. Only one third of the active physicians in the United States are family physicians, general internists, or general pediatricians, as compared with more than half of those in Canada and Western Europe" (Grumbach and Fry, 1993, p. 940).

At the time almost everyone agreed with this assessment. There was a mad scramble by hospitals and multispecialty clinics to acquire primary care practitioners. Several health plans, including Aetna and Prudential, developed their own primary care networks. A number of medical schools offered special incentives for physicians to select a primary care option for their advanced training.

It is our perception that in most markets the supply and demand for primary care services is in balance. How has this balance been achieved in such a short period of time? Here are several possible reasons:

- An increasing number of PCPs coming out of medical schools and advanced training
- An increasing number of physician's assistants and nurse practitioners performing tasks formerly carried out by PCPs
- Managed care backing off the primary care gatekeeper model, thus reducing the need for PCPs
- Developing evidence in some fields, such as cardiac care, that specialists are more cost effective and produce better clinical outcomes
- The capacity of PCPs and primary care networks to serve patients proving greater than anticipated
- A substantial number of specialists providing a significant amount of primary care

As we contemplated the supply and demand for PCPs in the context of the dramatic changes ahead (see the four scenarios in Chapter Thirteen), we concluded that some PCPs are at risk of not being able to continue to fulfill a need. For example, with increased emphasis on self-care and the use of the Internet, will the more sophisticated and higher-income consumers continue to rely on PCPs, or will they self-refer directly to specialists? In addition, people want choice in health care and dislike the gatekeeper concept. In other words the thinking of ten years ago about the critical role of PCPs may be changing—and changing dramatically.

Interspecialty Competition

The combination of the employer-based payment model and fragmentation among physicians has led to a health care system that is difficult to organize. Furthermore, the fact that many PCPs and specialists have not been able to work together in a managed care environment is disturbing. Part of the conflict is driven by the gate-keeper role that some health plans have asked PCPs to play. And then there is competition among the specialists.

Blair Tikker (1999), CEO of PhyLink, a physician network serving the southern part of the Denver area, contends, "Physicians are leveraging each other. This may be a bigger factor than health plan leveraging." Tikker is referring to physicians' fighting for capitated dollars and control over how health care is delivered. Many specialists resent the role of PCPs and do not respect the quality of care they deliver, particularly in cases where they believe that PCPs try to do too much. And there is plenty of competition among specialists for what they perceive to be a decreasing supply of health care dollars. PCPs resent what they perceive to be the "churning" of patients by some specialists—insisting on seeing the same patients over and over. PCPs are also concerned about not getting their patients back from specialists and not receiving reports on what services specialists have provided.

We observe competition among various medical specialties in many communities where the medical delivery system is fragmented—numerous solo practices and small groups and no dominating multispecialty groups. However, when we visit large, integrated systems led by multispecialty clinics, rivalry between PCPs and specialists is not an issue. There is mutual respect and a long history of collaboration.

A New Role for Primary Care Physicians?

We have believed for some time that the proper role of PCPs is that of coordinators of care, not gatekeepers. The gatekeeper concept has created problems for patients and PCPs and does not appear to have led to significant cost savings for payers or patients.

Bodenheimer, Bernard, and Casalino (1999) make a strong case that PCPs should be coordinators of care. As they put it, "The primary care coordination function can be explained using the analogy of the orchestra conductor. Conductors bring together individual musicians with diverse talents and meld them into a harmonious whole. If each musician simply played what he or she wished to play, the outcome would be sheer cacophony, even though each player might play exquisitely. The conductor allows the whole (an orchestra playing together) to be greater than the sum of the parts (the individual musicians)" (p. 2046).

Bodenheimer, Bernard, and Casalino note that for PCPs to play the coordinator role, there must be changes in incentives. First, patients should be charged higher copayments for uncoordinated visits to specialists. PCPs paid on a capitated or salaried basis should receive additional case management fees for complicated cases. Specialists should be paid on a salaried or capitated basis or, in the case of specialists who are not part of a system, on a contract capitation basis (a fixed sum for each referral).

In summary, we believe that for the most part there is a large and growing surplus of most types of physicians (primarily medical specialists but also PCPs) and hospital beds. Where do we go from here? Will we see more cardiologists driving taxis and an increasing number of hospitals converted to nursing homes or apartments?

Conclusions

Patrick Hays, former president and CEO of the national BCBS Association, believes that health plan mergers and acquisitions over the past few years have shifted the focus away from hospital consolidation. "But," Hays warns, "while the HMO industry diverts our attention, a larger trend that could further limit choices is bubbling below the surface: continuing consolidation among providers, particularly hospitals. In the long run, this development could prove more of a price pusher than most observers realize" (Hays, 1998, p. 2).

We believe Hays has a point, particularly with respect to the coming era, when consumers will want more choice. If hospital consolidation goes too far, choices will be limited. At the same time, however, we are concerned about the overzealous competition and duplication that often exist, especially in midsize communities where there are two or three hospitals.

Physician and medical group consolidation has been occurring at a steady pace over the past few years, and we believe this is positive for physicians and consumers. With an emphasis on clinical IT development, outcomes measurement, and the implementation of clinical guidelines, larger and better-organized groups of physicians have the best chance of adding value and finding ways to better serve patients.

There does not appear to be much question that in the first five years of the new millennium, all aspects of health care—health plans, hospitals, and medical groups—will move toward larger systems. Therefore, smaller, independent hospitals, solo practitioners or physicians in small groups, and start-up health plans will continue to face challenging times. There may be a few niche markets that certain physicians and hospitals can successfully serve, but this is unlikely to overcome the overall impact of a health care industry increasingly dominated by bigger players.

In Chapter Eleven we move on to a discussion of several major public policy issues in health care. The future of health care depends in large measure on how these issues are resolved.

The Effect of Changes in Public Policy

Policymaking is at least five years behind the realities of the health care market. . . . The trends toward consumerism and technology are not being adequately reflected in the thinking of policymakers and legislative leaders.

HEALTH CARE POLICY ADVISER

In our view, the U.S. health care system is unstable and headed for serious financial problems. A growing number of people who receive health care services are paying little or nothing (for example, the uninsured and Medicaid recipients), and the number of organizations and individuals paying the full tab is shrinking.

What are the major health care issues likely to affect physicians, hospitals, and other providers? Will the discussion of these policy issues take into account the growing roles of consumerism and technology? How will the resolution of these issues be reflected in the various scenarios of the future described in Chapter Thirteen? The major issues evaluated here are summarized in Exhibit 11.1.

A Look Back at How Policy Changes Have Affected Physicians and Hospitals

It is easy to be cynical about the minimal impact of past health care policy initiatives. However, despite the highly publicized failures of

Exhibit 11.1. Major Public Policy Issues Evaluated.

- Providing a payment source for uninsured Americans
- Ensuring solvency of the Medicare program
- Limiting the rate of increase in health care costs
- Financing new medical technology and drugs
- Reducing clinical variation
- Reorganizing systems of care to foster coordination
- Repositioning managed care for the future

the 1988 Medicare Catastrophic Coverage Act, which Congress repealed in 1989 following an uproar by seniors, and the 1993 Clinton reform efforts, there have been other important policy shifts and experiments led by federal and state governments.

Federal Policy Changes

As noted in Chapters One and Two, the Nixon administration's HMO initiatives in the 1970s, prospective payment (DRGs) in 1983, Medicare's RBRVS implemented in 1992, and the BBA of 1997 were notable federal efforts, and they all have had major impacts on health plans and providers.

On the legislative and regulatory front, laws governing private inurement (funds from not-for-profit systems going to for-profit entities or individuals), self-referral by physicians to laboratories and other facilities they own (Stark I and II), and antitrust have had important implications. The exemption of ambulatory surgery centers from the Stark rules has been followed by a rush by physicians to build these types of centers. The more recent efforts to attack fraud and abuse have had a profound impact: every organization has been forced to invest heavily in corporate compliance programs, and numerous medical groups and hospitals have been pressured into more conservative billing practices.

So if the future follows the past, as we look ahead at the likely changes in federal laws, rules, and regulations on health care, we can predict with a high degree of certainty that federal policies will have an important impact on health care financing and delivery.

The Clinton Reform Proposal

Despite the failure of the Clinton health care reform proposal, it had major effects. For example, the Clinton reform efforts focused on the needs and opportunities for providing health care over broader geographical areas, such as regions within a state or a state as a whole. The concept of accountable health plans caused many health care providers and health plans to expand their thinking in terms of relevant market areas, thus offering consumers in outlying areas more choice.

One interesting idea that came out of the Clinton reform proposal that has not been implemented is the concept of a standard benefits package. In fact, just the opposite has occurred. Health plans and the offerings of self-insured employers have become more diverse and customized to individual needs. It is not unusual for a moderately large health plan to offer more than one hundred variations of its basic product. Of course, more sophisticated information systems facilitate this kind of tailoring of health plans to the needs of specific small groups of people or even to individuals, and we expect even greater variety in the future.

We believe that the Clinton health care reform plan spurred development of PHOs and vertical integration strategies. For the more advanced integrated systems, there has been a major effort to provide coordinated, or "seamless," care for patients—certainly a worthwhile objective. The Clinton efforts also highlighted the role of PCPs.

So *even noteworthy failures have had a collective impact* on the way health care is financed and delivered in the United States. The debate of these ideas has a significant influence on hospital boards and other health care leaders and results in new thinking.

State Experiments

States also have substantial influence on health care policy through certificate-of-need laws, Medicaid reform initiatives, and other efforts. In the early to mid-1980s many states eliminated their certificate-of-need laws. The results have been mixed, with many states experiencing a boom in hospital construction. A sad by-product was the construction in the late-1980s of a number of behavioral health facilities, many of which have since closed and dragged old-line behavioral hospitals with them.

Probably the most notable state experiment in health care reform was the Oregon Medicaid waiver in the 1990s, which allowed the state to withhold dollars from very expensive procedures benefiting a small number of people in favor of serving a large number of children with basic primary care needs.

Hawaii has been a pacesetter in coming close to providing universal coverage. And a number of states—Tennessee, Montana, Texas, and others—have been leaders in adopting managed care principles to their Medicaid programs. Although these programs have produced mixed results, they have provided the opportunity to learn new ways to deal with the Medicaid population.

Major Public Policy Issues in Health Care

As we look ahead in the new century, we recognize that there are dozens of public policy issues relating to the future of how health care will be financed and delivered. Many of these issues, especially those surrounding the Medicare program and universal coverage, are being approached with a greater sense of urgency than at any time since 1993.

Our focus here is on issues that we believe will have the greatest impact on health care delivery and financing and on the adoption of technology and consumer choice. We do not address issues relating to consumer protection, such as the so-called patient's bill of rights. Part of the reason for not analyzing this group of issues is that we believe the strong trend toward consumerism in health care will largely render moot many of the concerns driving these issues. Another important public policy issue not analyzed here is the security of medical information. We believe that within five years this issue will be resolved and adequate safeguards will be provided to facilitate the development of the EMR.

Top Issues

Here are our nominees for the top health care issues that should dominate discussions during the first five years of the new millennium, ranked in order of priority:

1. *Providing a payment source for uninsured Americans.* As we discussed in Chapter Five, continuing to ignore the need for coverage for at least a portion of the uninsured population does not appear to be an option if we are to have an economically viable health care system. The cost shifting that results from the present system (over one-quarter of the population pays only a small fraction of the full cost of health care, and another major segment—Medicare recipients—can be expected to pay less than full costs) is threatening the stability of health care.

2. *Ensuring the solvency of the Medicare program.* This issue has also reached crisis proportions. Other than pouring in more money from projected federal "surpluses," most of the alternatives will be painful for consumers in terms of reduced benefits and to physicians, hospitals, and home health agencies in terms of reduced revenues.

3. *Limiting the rate of increase in health care costs.* The growth in health care costs, which affects employers and consumers as well as federal and state governments, has been on the back burner for the past five years. However, we see it coming to the forefront in a major way in the early part of the twenty-first century. An equally important issue will be establishing equity regarding who is paying and who is not.

4. *Financing new technology and drugs.* As discussed in Chapter Four, new technology and new drugs are leading the parade of factors driving health care costs. Even more important, economically feasible options for health plans and Medicare are limited. Will the purchase of new drugs be an individual responsibility, or will this coverage be included in Medicare and Medicaid? What are the arguments for a change in federal policy regarding the provision of prescription drug coverage by employers and health plans?

5. *Reducing clinical variation.* This is another way of discussing opportunities for improving quality. Despite the proliferation of clinical guidelines and the focus of national attention on this issue, it appears that little progress has been made in reducing clinical variation. In our view the extreme examples of clinical variation reflected in the *Dartmouth* small-area comparisons (Dartmouth Medical School, 1996) are a continuing embar-

rassment to everyone in health care and a major concern to
HCFA and others seeking ways to reduce health care costs.

6. *Reorganizing systems of care to focus on coordinated approaches.* The
present fee-for-service payment system used by HCFA leads to
fragmentation rather than coordinated care for the chronically
ill, a large group who account for a substantial proportion of
all health care spending. What can be done to align the financial incentives in Medicare funding with the needs of those
with chronic diseases?

7. *Repositioning managed care for the future.* Is managed care capable of making the needed changes to reposition itself for the
future? What policy changes are needed to make managed
care more consumer and physician friendly and politically
viable?

Several of these issues are interrelated. The ways in which new
technology and prescription drugs are financed (for example,
whether included in health plan and Medicare benefits packages
or paid for out of pocket) will affect the prospects for long-term
solvency of Medicare. Improving quality of care by reducing clinical variation and coordinating care for chronically ill patients
should also have significant cost impact, especially for the Medicare
program.

Discussion of the Major Issues

Our discussion and preliminary analysis of major issues is intended
to help frame the four scenarios presented in Chapter Thirteen.

Issue 1: A Payment Source for the Uninsured

Some refer to this as *universal coverage.* Universal coverage is often
confused with a single-payer system; however, we are using the term
universal coverage more narrowly to mean a payment source, or
combination of sources, for the uninsured (the CHIPS program,
for example, or such measures as improving Medicaid or allowing
those between the ages of fifty-five and sixty-four to purchase
Medicare coverage).

The urgency of the problem prompted two political opponents to join in calling for progress in helping the growing number of uninsured Americans: "Too often, when Congress turns to health issues, it ends up applying legislative Band-Aids. It's time to address underlying causes. The biggest health problem facing the country is the uninsured" (Armey and Stark, 1999).

Uninsured and Medicaid Populations

At the time of the 1993 debate on the Clinton health care proposal, there were an estimated thirty-seven million Americans who lacked health insurance. We project that the number of uninsured surpassed forty-five million in 2000. This means that the uninsured have been increasing at the rate of more than one million a year, and this has been happening in a favorable economic climate. See Figure 11.1 for our estimates of the composition of the uninsured population in 2000.

Figure 11.1. Distribution of the Uninsured, 2000.

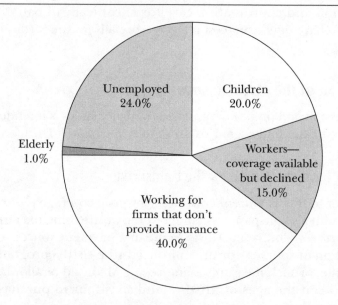

Sources: Kaiser Family Foundation; National Coalition on Healthcare; Health Insurance Association of America; authors' estimates.

Without some reform in the health care system, the number of uninsured can be expected to reach fifty-five million (18 percent of all Americans) by 2005. With a recession the number of uninsured would almost certainly exceed sixty million.

Myth: The Uninsured Receive Adequate Health Care

"Almost everyone we see has a story which illustrates, sometimes tragically, the plight of the uninsured," says Robert Le Bow, physician and medical director of the Terry Reilly Health Center, a community clinic in Nampa, Idaho. "We're talking dead mothers because they couldn't afford prenatal care, or diabetes wildly out of control, for lack of simple medications" (Quinn, 1999, p. 49). On a more quantitative basis the Kaiser Family Foundation (1999) reports these findings:

- One in five uninsured children have no regular source of care, and uninsured children are 30 percent more likely to fall behind on well-child care and 80 percent more likely never to have had routine care.
- Uninsured children are at least 70 percent more likely than insured children not to have received medical care for common conditions like asthma—illnesses that, if left untreated, can lead to more serious health problems.
- Over half of uninsured adults have no regular source of care. Fifty-five percent of uninsured adults say they have postponed getting care, and a quarter have not filled a prescription in the past year—because they could not afford it.

Poor Quality of Care for the Uninsured

Donna Shalala (1999, p. 47), secretary of health and human services, says, "At the top, ours is the best health care in the world. . . . At the low end, though, our system can be lousy, particularly for people who are not treated early enough." The following story about patient dumping illustrates another part of the problem of the uninsured:

> [Colorado] House lawmakers heard shocking tales Wednesday of patients with broken bones, heart-attack symptoms and tubal pregnancies being denied appropriate treatment because of their lack of insurance.

University Hospital President Dennis Brimhall testified about his concerns over the practice of "patient dumping" before a state legislative committee Wednesday morning, reading from a list of emergency-room patients he said his hospital immediately admitted who had been turned away from other hospitals and doctors' offices.

Brimhall stunned several lawmakers with one case he related in which a woman had "fetal demise"—she was carrying a dead fetus—for several days and was having a hard time finding someone in the health-care community to treat her.

Brimhall went on to say that a number of people with serious illnesses and injuries were falling through the cracks because private physicians would not care for them. "There are patients getting care that we would be embarrassed about," Brimhall said [Johnston, 1999, p. A4].

A Financial Crisis Is Brewing

In our view few factors are as important for the future of the U.S. health care system as focusing on the problem of providing a reasonable payment source for a significant portion of the uninsured. The stability of the health care system is at stake.

The high proportion of nonpayers and deep discounters (Medicare appears to be moving in this direction) is rapidly destabilizing the health care system by placing too much of a burden on the other payers, primarily individuals and employers. Because of its size, Medicare dictates price, paying an amount determined by averages and politics. Other than individuals and employers, who is left to pick up the shortfall?

Although cost shifting takes place in almost any industry, the magnitude of this practice in health care has become increasingly large and destabilizing. As indicated by our analysis in Chapter Five, the problem is reaching crisis proportions.

Cost of Providing Universal Coverage May Be Manageable

We do not accept the argument that the cost of providing coverage for the uninsured would be exorbitant. We are essentially talking about the need for access to primary care, and these types of services represent less than 5 percent of all health care costs. (As noted in Chapter Three, physician services are about 20 percent of all health care spending, and we estimate that primary care is a quarter of this.) With 16 percent of the U.S. population uninsured, the total cost of providing universal coverage for primary care services should not exceed 1 percent of total health care spending, or about $13 billion in 2000.

What About More Serious Illnesses?

The uninsured tend to wait until they are more seriously ill and then visit an emergency room or show up at a specialist's office. Both of these alternatives are expensive, and physicians and hospitals bear most of the cost. Almost everyone agrees that the uninsured do not use the health care system appropriately. Use of hospitals and specialists should decline with more ready access to primary care. This would mean of course that with some form of universal coverage many physicians and nearly all hospitals would not have to pass along the cost of caring for the uninsured to other payers.

Who Would Pay for Universal Coverage?

It is obvious, based on the failed efforts of the Clinton reform proposal (and the "Harry and Louise" ads aired by the health insurance industry), that it will not happen if employers are asked to pick up the tab. In fact, the Health Insurance Association of America has come out in favor of a federally funded program to cover most of the uninsured. A *New York Times* article reported, "The insurance companies also proposed a new Government subsidy, in the form of vouchers, for uninsured people between 100 percent and 200 percent of the poverty level. The vouchers, about $2,000 a year for each person, could be used to buy private health insurance of the type sold by members of the association" (Pear, 1999a, p. Y16).

Incremental Approaches May Be More Politically and Economically Realistic

Another approach, advocated by David Blumenthal of Massachusetts General Hospital, would be to focus on three groups for which it may be more realistic to obtain public agreement and support for insurance coverage: the ten million children, three million persons between the ages of fifty-five and sixty-four, and employed adults with incomes of up to 200 percent of the poverty level (Blumenthal, 1999). "From the standpoint of administrative simplicity," Blumenthal maintains, "all three groups could be covered under existing Medicaid and Medicare programs. Children and the working poor or nearly poor could be covered by expanding eligibility for Medicaid, and older Americans could be given the opportunity to buy into the Medicare program through a federal subsidy proportional to their income."

Another alternative is to expand the public health system, including increased funding for community health centers. Based on our experience, these centers provide valued health care services to a significant number of individuals and at relatively low cost.

Even if the problem is attacked on an incremental basis, it would lead to meaningful reductions in the number of uninsured Americans. This issue has been off the radar screen too long, and as a result, both the public and the health care system have become complacent. However, continuing to ignore the problem is not a realistic option.

In Chapter Thirteen, which proposes four scenarios for the future of health care, we anticipate little or no progress on this issue in scenarios 1 (incremental change) and 2 (constrained resources). Scenario 4 contains elements of the AMA's proposal for individual insurance, and this would include substantial progress in reducing the number of the uninsured through tax deductions and credits.

Issue 2: Medicare Solvency

This is also an issue of vital importance, not only to the more than forty million Medicare beneficiaries and their families but also to employers and workers who continue to pay the lion's share of the cost of this federal program. Of course, everyone is concerned about the financial impact of the baby boomers, expected to hit around 2010, and the resulting drop in the number of workers available to support each Medicare recipient.

Impact on Hospitals

The impact of the BBA is creating especially serious problems for hospitals. Don Wilson, president of the Kansas Hospital Association, told us that when he and twenty-seven hospital CEOs visited their senators and congressional representatives, "our messages this year to members of our state delegation were loud and clear: *no more cuts* and *fix the balanced budget act.*" A letter to Senator Pete Domenici, chairman of the budget committee, written by Senator Pat Roberts of Kansas (Feb. 8, 1999), said that 56 percent of Kansas hospitals were already losing money on their Medicare patients and every hospital in the state was losing money on Medicare out-patient services.

Policy Options

There are many alternatives for improving the prospects of Medicare solvency, including shifting funds from the so-called fed-eral budget surplus (as advocated by President Clinton in 1999), gradually increasing the Medicare eligibility age to sixty-seven (fol-lowing the same schedule as previously approved for Social Secu-rity), and shifting to a premium support system similar to defined contributions (discussed in Chapter Twelve).

Premium Support

The chairman of the National Bipartisan Commission on the Future of Medicare, Senator John Breaux of Louisiana, has been a strong proponent of premium support. In reporting on the results of the commission's efforts, *The Economist* asked, "Why not give the elderly vouchers—premium support—so that they can shop around for the most appropriate health plan? As Robert Moffit, of the right-wing Heritage Foundation, argues, this approach is already used by the Federal Employees Health Benefits Programme, and so should be good enough to be extended generally" ("Medicare Reform: Promises, Promises," 1999, p. 32). In response Representative Sher-rod Brown, a Democrat from Ohio, said, "The idea that vouchers will empower seniors to choose a health plan that best suits their needs is quite simply a myth. The reality is that seniors will be forced to accept whatever plan they can afford" (p. 32).

With premium support Medicare recipients living in larger markets would have the ability to choose from a variety of types of health plans—HMOs, PPOs, and traditional fee-for-service arrange-ments. Those Medicare participants desiring a more expensive plan would pay the extra cost out of their pockets. (Of course, there are no assurances that competing plans would be available in smaller markets or that these plans would be interested in competing for Medicare business.)

Other Possible Changes in Medicare

From a political viewpoint the changes being considered that might reduce costs have to be weighed against the need to maintain or improve benefits. On the latter point these benefits might be expanded to include outpatient drug coverage (discussed later in this chapter). Another issue affecting costs is the desire to allow persons who are on Social Security but between the ages of fifty-five and sixty-four (often early retirees) to purchase Medicare coverage. This would reduce the number of the uninsured.

In our view the movement toward premium support makes sense and is consistent with the way many Americans are likely to be purchasing health plan coverage in the future. Therefore when individuals move into the Medicare program, the change would be less dramatic.

Issue 3: Controlling Costs and Achieving Financial Equity

In Chapter Three we noted that health care costs in the United States are substantially higher than in any other country in the world. In Chapter Four we analyzed the forces driving year-to-year increases in health care spending and forecasted the annual rates of increase in health care spending for the first five years of the new century—it is not a pretty picture. Without universal coverage these increasing costs will be borne by a smaller and smaller number of payers, primarily employers and individuals. What can be done to slow the growth of health care costs and achieve more equity in the system?

Cost Containment Opportunities

Efforts on the part of medical groups, hospitals, integrated systems, and health plans to reduce clinical variation through clinical information technology, clinical guidelines, and outcomes measurement should eventually contribute to lowering annual health care spending increases. Most health care organizations are engaged in performance improvement projects aimed at increasing their efficiency and cutting costs. But will these be sufficient to ensure the economic viability of major segments of the health care industry? With all of the other upward pressures on costs—new technology and drugs, aging of the population, surplus of medical specialists, inconsistent reimbursement models—it is doubtful.

Increasing Demand for Services

The other side of the trend toward consumerism is that consumer demand for health care services is increasing. (We define *demand* as the combination of a perceived need or desire for a product plus the ability to pay.) The evidence considered in Chapters Six and Seven indicates that many upper-income consumers are willing and able to pay more out of their pockets for health care services. If the economy remains strong, personal incomes continue to grow in real terms, the stock and bond markets remain at high levels, consumer confidence remains high, and some progress is made in solving the problem of the uninsured, there is a high probability that consumers will spend more out of their pockets for both clinically necessary and lifestyle drugs, diagnostic and clinical procedures (such as cosmetic surgery, in vitro fertilization, laser eye surgery, knee and hip replacement), medical devices (such as high-tech hearing aids), and complementary and alternative medicines. This is reflected in scenario 4 in Chapter Thirteen.

Health Care Spending as a Percentage of Gross Domestic Product

Despite the protests of consumers and the growing objections of employers and government payers, we believe that health care spending, after adjustments for inflation and figured on a per capita basis, will continue to increase. We projected in Chapter Four that the proportion of GDP spent on health care will reach 15 percent by 2005.

Leland Kaiser, a health care futurist, told us that he expects health care spending to eventually reach 22 to 25 percent of GDP and that he does not see a problem with this possibility. "Health care is bigger and more important than most people realize," Kaiser said. "Also, U.S. health care providers are increasingly offering their services to people from around the world. Health care is on the verge of becoming one of our biggest export industries" (interview, Mar. 31, 1999).

We think the *fairness* of the system in terms of who is paying for health care compared with who is benefiting is a potentially more explosive issue than the level of health care spending as a percentage of GDP. The system is becoming increasingly inequitable, and we do not believe employers and consumers will stand for it much longer. This means of course that the United States has to move toward offering universal coverage and that both the public and private sectors must pay their fair share.

Issue 4: Financing Drugs and Advances in Medical Technology

Most Americans are in favor of the development and application of medical technology and new, improved drugs. Who would not be in favor of laparoscopic surgery for the removal of a gallbladder compared with an eight-inch incision? The dramatic improvements in surgical techniques to remove cataracts continue to be a blessing for millions. The increased ability to replace hips and knees has been a boon to many hundreds of thousands of Americans. Arthroscopic knee surgery has extended the careers of many athletes.

Most Americans look forward to a flow of new drugs and are anxiously awaiting other new pharmaceutical products that promise to relieve chronic conditions like arthritis, asthma, macular degeneration of the eyes, high blood pressure, and diabetes. Breakthroughs in drugs effective in treating heart disease, cancer, Alzheimer's disease, and AIDS are widely anticipated.

Consumers Need Access to New Drugs

It is difficult to argue against the proposition that drugs are an integral part of the care of most diseases and that without access to prescription drugs, health care spending will be even higher and human suffering far worse. Stephen Soumerai, chairman of Harvard University's Drug Policy Research Institute, says that elderly people who do not get sufficient medication often get too sick to stay independent and end up in the hospital or nursing home. He said, "Drugs are the glue that holds the medical system together. We can't afford not to cover people with chronic illnesses, or whose independence rests on access to medications" (Lagnado, 1998, p. A1).

The implications of not offering financial assistance for out-patient drug coverage would be severe. For example, Nancy Whitelaw and Gail Warden of the Henry Ford Health System in Detroit point out that persons sixty-five years of age and older consume more than one-third of all prescription drugs—an average of fourteen prescriptions per person per year (Whitelaw and Warden, 1999). "Delivery systems are incapable of carrying this financial burden alone," Whitelaw and Warden assert, "but we cannot provide effective health care to persons with chronic disease who cannot obtain a regular supply of appropriate medications" (pp. 135–136).

It is not unusual for an elderly couple to spend $500 a month or more for drugs and related health care products. An excerpt from *USA Today* provides an example: "For Ned Cook at the Pascal Senior Center (Glen Burnie, Maryland), the insulin his wife injects for her diabetes costs $22 a bottle; she needs four to six bottles a month. He carries a small notebook with a handwritten list of the medications they each take: eight for him; 11 for her. For a time, he tried to finance the purchases on their credit cards, but with debts of $15,000 the cards have been cut off" (Welch and Page, 1999, p. A2).

As two researchers from Harvard Medical School advise, "Restricted coverage for needed drugs may be a false economy. A follow-up study in New Hampshire found that chronically ill elderly persons affected by limits on Medicaid drug payments were twice as likely as members of a control cohort to enter nursing homes, where they remained permanently in most cases. Increased nursing home and hospital stays during the 11 months the cap was in effect cost Medicaid more than the program saved in drug expenditures" (Soumerai and Ross-Degnan, 1999, p. 727).

How to Finance Drug Coverage?

The issue, then, is how to pay for all the wonderful new medical technology and the increasingly sophisticated drugs. Given the staggering problems of financing Medicare and Medicaid and the cost issues inevitably facing employers, we see no alternative but for consumers to pay for at least a portion of the cost of drugs. Some outpatient drugs will undoubtedly become part of Medicare's benefit package, but on financial grounds it will be increasingly tough to justify their inclusion without strict limits and some additional financial contributions by participants.

How Will the Situation Play Out?

As noted earlier and discussed in more detail in Chapter Twelve, an increasing number of Americans are likely to receive defined contributions for their health benefits. They will select the plan that most meets their needs and fits their budgets. Individuals concerned about the high cost of drugs may select a plan that pays a high percentage of the cost of drugs and less for other services. For example, they may choose plans with higher copayments and deductibles for primary care services and better coverage for drugs and more catastrophic events.

We do not believe that expanded drug benefits should be tacked onto Medicare or managed care plans without some added payment by consumers. Consumers will have to make a choice, and that is what consumer-driven health care will be all about in the early part of the new century.

Issue 5: Improving Quality of Care

The more we work in health care, the more we realize that the variations in clinical practice patterns and quality are greater than we may have thought a few years earlier. The differences among the best physicians and medical groups compared with those that are average or below average are not marginal; they are significant.

Kate Paul, former western regional president for Kaiser Permanente, when asked a question about the biggest issue facing managed care, replied that it was the industry's "not absolutely knowing what quality is and what quality isn't. A lot of what's done to and for patients is not done on the basis of evidence but is rather done on the basis of the way physicians were trained. Because we've got lots of different doctor schools and lots of different theories, people are trained and oriented in different directions. That causes a great deal of ambiguity and difference of opinion about what quality is and what quality isn't" (Conklin, 1999).

Small Area Studies

John Wennberg and his associates at Dartmouth (Dartmouth Medical School, 1996) summarize it this way: "Health services researchers have long been aware of large variations in the use of medical care among communities and regions. In the 1930s, the British pediatrician J. Allison Glover observed that the rates of surgical removal of the tonsils in British schoolchildren varied widely, depending on the district in which the students lived and the school health doctors who examined them. In some school districts, more than 50% of children had tonsillectomies, while in others, less than 10% did" (p. 2).

Moving to more recent years, Wennberg's report says, "In the 1980s, a series of studies of Boston and New Haven, Connecticut, extended insights in the variation phenomenon, demonstrating once again that in health care markets, geography is destiny: the care one receives depends in large part on the supply of resources available in the place where one lives—and the practice patterns of local physicians" (p. 2). Later studies show the same patterns of huge variations among adjoining communities with similar demographic characteristics. The availability of physicians (mainly specialists) and hospital beds appears to be the dominant factor determining clinical variation.

Different Definitions of Quality

In consumer and physician research we have conducted over the years, we have found major differences between the way consumers define quality of care and the way physicians see quality. Physicians give more weight to the technical qualifications of other physicians, their reputations, board certification, professional accomplishments, and past training. Consumers look at "bedside manner," promptness, meeting commitments, and friendliness of staff. With increased use of patient satisfaction surveys, we suspect that physicians, not consumers, will be changing their views about what constitutes quality.

What Can Be Done to Reduce Clinical Variation?

Reducing clinical variation continues to be a challenge for physicians. Increased use of clinical guidelines, outcomes measures, and databases made possible by information systems development all add up to significant opportunities to improve clinical quality of care in the years ahead. We believe that health care quality will improve most rapidly when consumers demand it. The fragmented employer-based system, combined with Medicare and its emphasis on fee-for-service payment, are unlikely to lead to significant quality improvements.

Looking ahead, we believe that quality of care will be the highest in scenario 4, the combination of a consumer- and technology-driven health care system. Therefore policy initiatives that favor the development of this scenario (such as changing the tax code to encourage individually purchased health insurance and reducing the number of the uninsured) should lead to quality improvements on a substantial scale.

Issue 6: Reorganizing Medicare to Provide More Coordinated Systems of Care for the Chronically Ill

Nancy Whitelaw and Gail Warden of the Henry Ford Health System say that "Medicare is organized around a set of principles that are fundamentally inflationary and frustrate efforts to improve the health status of the elderly. There must be a willingness to risk parting with what we know does not work and to build organizational and payment systems based on coordinated systems of care and chronic disease management" (1999, pp. 141–142).

Whitelaw and Warden point out that the dominant health problems of Medicare recipients are chronic illness: "88 percent of all Medicare beneficiaries have at least one chronic condition" (p. 138). They say that, generally, "less attention is needed on how to reduce inpatient days; more study is required on how to provide high-quality care in the most appropriate setting at the optimal time" (p. 134). They go on to say Medicare policy reinforces fragmentation and a focus on hospitals rather than care for those with chronic illnesses.

Bruce Clark, senior vice president of Age Wave Health Services, a California company that provides connections with mature consumers, says essentially the same thing: "The problem is that as our population ages, Medicare is becoming increasingly irrelevant to the genuine needs of the population it is designed to serve. We are spending money in the wrong places. . . . Today we have 34 million people over the age of 65, and on average they are treating and managing three to four chronic conditions each over the span of decades. As a result, the things millions of seniors really need to manage their health are not even addressed by Medicare" (Walker, 1998, p. 6).

In another example of the discontinuities associated with Medicare, a growing number of long-term care facilities are denying access to hospitalized patients, especially those who depend on ventilators or need intravenous drug therapy, kidney dialysis, or tracheotomy care. The problem is at least partially related to payment rates. Administrators of nursing facilities report that reduced federal reimbursement resulting from the BBA does not cover the cost of care for patients with complicated needs. As one article comments, "The trend shows how squeezing on part of the health-care sector can have an unintended impact on another" (McGinley, 1999, p. B1).

This is borne out by our interviews with hospital and health system leaders. One hospital CEO in a western state told us that nursing homes in the area are reluctant to accept Medicare patients whom the hospital wants to discharge. "Our average length of stay has increased by one day over the past six months," the CEO said. "I believe this is one of the unintended consequences of the BBA."

We agree with Whitelaw, Warden, Clark, and the hospital CEO: our experience in performing community health care needs assessments has shown that senior medical care and support systems are often weak or lacking. More recently, cuts in Medicare reimbursement for very ill patients have made things even more complicated. This is the area where most of the unmet community needs fall.

Although an increasing number of industry experts are recognizing this as a problem, we have not heard much discussion about, or many specific proposals for, changing Medicare to deal with the issue. However, we expect progress over the next five years, perhaps involving greater use of what we have learned from disease management programs for chronic illnesses.

Issue 7: Can Managed Care Be Reformed?

Dan Callahan, cofounder of the Hastings Center, which focuses on biomedical ethics, asked this question during a Harvard roundtable discussion ("The Future of Health Care," 1999, p. 50): "Is managed care capable, over the long run, of reforming itself—for instance, giving physicians enough time with their patients, as well as giving patients some choice? The question I put to Mr. Huber [head of Aetna] is, right now there are lots of problems: you have the mandate problem on the one hand, you have excessive demands—the unwillingness of people to give up anything—on the other. Is managed care reformable in principle, even if we don't in practice know exactly what to do tomorrow?"

Richard Huber responded by saying that managed care is a young industry that is continuing to transform itself. "The amateur hour is over. Oxford and a number of other innovative managed-care companies were founded by visionary, charismatic entrepreneurs, and that worked very well during the first phase of the industry. The industry changed" (p. 50).

Huber went on to say that managed care has been through two phases and that there are two more to come. The first phase was switching from buying retail to buying wholesale. "We're in the second phase now," Huber explained, "which is managing utilization, managing the most absurd types of utilization—the MRI for the ingrown toenail" (p. 50). This was Huber's description of the third and fourth phases: "The third phase, which we're moving into now, is increasing disease management: using the data we have access to, converting that data into meaningful information, and then doing something about it. The fourth phase, which I alluded to early on, is when we really begin to apply standards and true performance measurements to this huge industry, and try to implement the best practices" (p. 50).

In considering the future of managed care, we believe that Huber's vision of phases three and four makes sense. However, we believe that subsequent phases of managed care are likely to involve several additional challenges:

- Learning how to market to consumers and purchasing alliances rather than employers.
- Finding a financial incentive system for physicians other than capitated payment of PCPs. Capitation does not work in many parts of the country (see Chapter Twelve).
- Developing the IT systems to be able to more readily assess the diagnosis and treatment of patients by physicians, including an increased emphasis on evidence-based medicine.

- Improving services and convenience and making the whole system more patient friendly.
- Continuing to offer consumers the freedom to choose physicians and hospitals and still controlling health care costs. The discussion earlier in this chapter and in Chapter Ten about the potential role of PCPs as coordinators of care could contribute to the resolution of this issue.

Huber characterized managed care as a young industry. Although it is young in terms of number of years in the marketplace, *we view managed care as a mature industry* with a tremendous infrastructure built around a business-as-usual view of the future. Therefore, shifting gears in ways that will enable managed care to make meaningful changes and continue to be viable will be difficult.

Repairing relationships with physicians and medical groups will be a continuing challenge, as will the current approach of competing based on the health status of individuals and groups (such as by cherry picking). The challenges of reconfiguring managed care are enormous, and public policy considerations of the future of managed care should be moving the debate in this direction.

Conclusions

Part of the problem in thinking about major public policy issues is considering them on the basis of the old paradigm in health care—a continuation of the employer-based system with an emphasis on defined benefits. We believe that when growth in consumerism and technology are factored in, several of these issues will be resolved.

One policy analyst in Washington, D.C., told us, "Many of the issues we are considering are based on health care the way it was ten years ago. It makes me sick. Sometimes I want to get up and walk out of meetings on this subject." Her point was that there is the need to envision a health care system where consumerism and technology are increasingly important and to make policy decisions based on the best ways to direct these twin forces.

Health care has simply become too large and important for those in the federal government, large employers, or drug companies to dictate the rules. Like it or not, *consumers* are going to decide with their dollars and their feet how to allocate resources among various health care alternatives and other possible expenditures. As we noted at the beginning of this chapter, this is one of the reasons we have not discussed proposals for a patient's bill of rights; by 2005, we believe, in a future dominated by consumers and technology, these kinds of issues will become irrelevant.

As for how the important policy issues discussed in this chapter will be resolved and how they will affect health care in the future, here are our bets on what will happen over the first five years of the new millennium:

- There will be incremental progress in reducing the number of the uninsured, but universal coverage will remain an elusive goal. (This is consistent with scenarios 3 and 4 in Chapter Thirteen.)
- Funding for Medicare will be increased above the levels spelled out in the BBA of 1997, with relief for a number of health care sectors, especially rehabilitation and teaching hospitals. Although not always agreeing with relaxing the BBA, nearly all of the health care policy analysts we contacted agreed that this would happen.
- Little progress will be made in controlling the expected $100 billion per year increase in health care costs. Unless there is an economic recession (scenario 2), the forces driving these costs are virtually unstoppable.
- Financing for new drugs and technological advances will largely be left up to consumers. Consumers will either pay for desirable new drugs and technology out of their pockets or change the type of health insurance they buy (purchasing, for example, less first-dollar coverage and more catastrophic coverage that would include expensive drugs and medical technology).
- There is a long way to go in improving quality and reducing clinical variation, but progress is coming. Clinical information systems, guidelines, and outcomes measures will be major contributors to improved quality and service. The threat of medical malpractice is already encouraging the development and use of clinical guidelines.

- Reorganizing Medicare to provide a more coordinated approach to the management of chronic diseases will be difficult to achieve. We believe that if Medicare payment were shifted to a voucher or premium support model, there would be a better chance of this happening.

Chapter Twelve

The Potential of Different Payment System Models

The current pattern—shifting of costs to employees, paring of benefits, and resulting increases in the number of the uninsured and underinsured—is likely to persist as long as the basic system of employer-provided health insurance continues.

ROBERT KUTTNER, "The American Health Care System: Employer-Sponsored Health Coverage," *New England Journal of Medicine,* 1999

Stating his dissatisfaction with managed care and the employer-based system, Arnold Relman, editor-in-chief emeritus of the *New England Journal of Medicine,* responded to the question, "Why are you so sure that managed care is doomed?" Relman's answer: "The present system [of managed care] simply isn't viable. It pits the interest of the insurer against that of the patient, and it ensnares and infuriates the medical profession. Doctors, nurses and others cannot do things the way they were trained and know to be the best way" (Gorner, 1998). Reflecting another viewpoint, Roger Gilbertson, CEO of MeritCare in Fargo, North Dakota, told us, "Health care is too fragmented. It is too compartmentalized. Patients get lost in this thing." We could quote many others with different views on various health care payment models and how payment needs to be changed in the future.

The primary purpose of this chapter is to review a number of alternative payment models that most affect employers, Medicare, and consumers. We also discuss capitation versus fee-for-service, with an emphasis on how these two payment methods are likely to relate to physicians and hospitals in the future.

Payment System Models of the Future: Overview

There are a number of possible alternative models of how the health care payment system might develop over the first five years of the new century (see Figure 12.1). For purposes of analysis and developing scenarios for the future, we believe there are five fairly broad potential models, each reflecting where health care payment might be headed:

1. *Continuation of employer-based model.* This alternative includes the continued maturing, or "graying," of managed care. It would include more mandates and regulations and legislation aimed at increasing patients' rights. Managed care growth would slow because the commercial market is saturated, and there would be continuing difficulties—mainly poor reimbursement—in extending this type of health plan to the Medicare population.
2. *Managed care is invigorated.* Under this alternative, HCFA would find ways to make Medicare risk products more attractive to physician groups, hospitals, and health plans and put some steam back into the growth of Medicare HMOs. This alternative also includes additional Medicaid beneficiaries moving into managed care and added coverage of children in the combined federal-state CHIPS program.
3. *Increased emphasis on defined contributions rather than defined benefits.* Different people have different names for this trend. In the context of Medicare it is referred to as "premium support" rather than a system that pays for all defined benefits. It means that an increasing number of employees or those on Medicare and Medicaid will receive a fixed amount of money per month to cover health care services, and it will be up to these individuals to make decisions on which health plans and benefit packages they want.
4. *MSAs and vouchers.* A form of vouchers is being used by the Buyer's Health Care Action Group (BHCAG) in the Twin Cities. In addition to growth in vouchers this alternative would

include more widespread use of MSAs. Both vouchers and MSAs give consumers more control over health care decision making and more financial responsibility.

5. *Individual health insurance substitutes for the employer-based payment system.* In mid-1998 the AMA proposed that the United States shift away from the employer-based health care system to one in which consumers play a more direct role. The AMA's proposed alternative is similar to the Heritage Foundation consumer choice model that initially surfaced prior to the Clinton health care reform proposal discussions and received serious consideration in several states, including Maryland. Both models include tax incentives, including tax credits, for the uninsured to purchase health plan coverage.

We have not included a Canadian-style single-payer system among the payment models described and assessed in this chapter. Despite 1999 studies sponsored by the Massachusetts Medical Society showing renewed interest in a single-payer system, we detect little or no national support for this model and believe that the odds are stacked against enactment of a single-payer system, especially during the five-year time frame used in this book.

Continuation of Employer-Based Model

With 85 percent market penetration among employees working for firms that offer health insurance coverage, HMOs and PPOs have limited growth potential in the commercial sector. *Managed care is a mature industry* in the more heavily populated areas of the country.

Under this model we expect open-access or POS plans to continue to be popular. In a sense these types of plans represent a step back from the trend toward more tightly managed care that developed from the time of inception of HMOs through the early 1990s. With the employer-based model, we anticipate greater use of disease management programs (for such illnesses as diabetes, asthma, congestive heart failure, and arthritis, for example). These efforts are proving to be cost effective for health plans and increasingly valued by both employers and participants.

Figure 12.1. Continuum of Payment System Models.

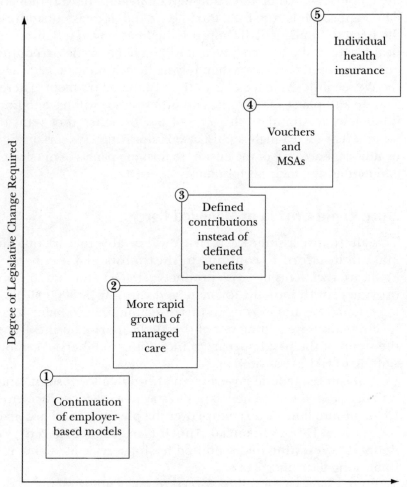

A federally mandated patient's bill of rights would be part of the employer-based model. Although we believe this sort of mandated approach is "too little too late" in that it does not address the need to fundamentally improve the financing and delivery of health care in the United States, it will increasingly be part of the employer-based payment system relying heavily on managed care.

We see little evidence of growth in capitated payment. Therefore, health plans, employers, and other payers will have to find other ways to stimulate the type of performance they want to achieve. The increasingly sophisticated information systems of large health plans are part of the answer to forming panels of physicians and monitoring their performance.

More Rapid Growth of Managed Care

This alternative assumes that HCFA will be able to work out the kinks in its efforts to continue to shift substantial numbers of Medicare recipients into risk products (HMOs) and that this will provide growth impetus for managed care. As of 2000 HCFA's experience was not moving in this direction; that is, many large health plans were getting out of the Medicare risk business, and the trend of the past few years of increasing numbers of seniors shifting to HMOs was slowing.

But can the federal government afford to allow a substantial number of Medicare beneficiaries to stay in a fee-for-service environment with little or no control over the physicians and hospitals used? Given HCFA's financial crunch (see Chapter Eleven), we doubt that reverting to discounted fee-for-service medicine is a viable long-term alternative.

In our view HCFA will be forced to make adjustments in the monthly payment rates for Medicare HMOs, primarily in rural counties where the rates are typically below national averages. Increased rates in metropolitan areas also will have to be sufficient to induce health plans to continue to offer Medicare risk products and for seniors to find it advantageous to give up the freedom of choice they now enjoy in favor of Medicare HMOs. All of this will have to occur if total HMO enrollment is to exceed one hundred million Americans by 2005.

Defined Contribution Rather Than Defined Benefits

We introduced the concept of defined contributions in Chapter Six as evidence of the trend toward consumers taking control of health care. Here is additional background, both pro and con, about defined contributions (or *premium support*—the term used in a Medicare context).

A Business Perspective

In an article reviewing the past twenty-five years of the influential Washington Business Group on Health, much of the concern was about defined contributions and the ability of employees and their families to become informed consumers. "When you talk about defined contribution in the future it would suggest that there must be some steps that move us toward becoming informed users," explains Sue Nelson of Texas Instruments (Reese, 1999, p. 32).

A human resources expert expresses skepticism about defined contributions: Today's market is set up to address the needs of employers, not individuals. Consequently, the delivery system isn't conducive to patients searching for a plan on their own. Bruce Taylor of GTE said, "One of the problems with moving to that kind of model is you haven't got an organized way for people to buy effectively. . . . If you just toss all the people that we have out into the marketplace, they would have a great deal of difficulty affording, purchasing, deciding. It would be a free-for-all, and it would be very ugly. So I don't know if it's realistic right now to say that's an alternative" (Reese, 1999, pp. 32–33).

"All of the pieces aren't in place to make that play out robustly right now," says Chuck Buck, project leader for health care quality and strategic initiatives at General Electric (Reese, 1999, p. 33). But defined contributions fit the long-term vision of a more consumer-focused health care system at all levels that would focus on "choice of plans, choice of doctors, [and] choice of treatments," as Sue Nelson says. "I think we're all supportive of that in a broad concept," she concludes (Reese, 1999, p. 33).

The AMA proposal, discussed later in this chapter, includes defined contributions by employers as one of the three main features of its plan. The AMA also supports the concept of purchasing coalitions for consumers (American Medical Association, 1999b).

Importance of Purchasing Organizations

Bill Lindsay, president of Benefit Management & Design in Denver, agrees that for either defined contribution or individual insurance plans to work, there would have to be effective consumer purchasing alliances in place. "This is absolutely critical," Lindsay believes. "Asking consumers to purchase their own insurance without some form of purchasing alliance would put individuals at the mercy of health plans, and they would have no bargaining power" (interview, July 21, 1999). Lindsay also said the federal government needs to take the lead in facilitating the formation of consumer purchasing alliances.

It is also possible that some large retail chains might take on the role of purchasing agent for customers or members. We are aware of at least two national retailers that are seriously considering adding health plans to their range of products and services.

Defined Contributions for Retiree Health Benefits

IBM and other large companies are using a defined-contribution approach to limiting their liabilities for retiree health costs. These are referred to as "health cash accounts." Employers offering these accounts deposit annual credits in defined-contribution-type plans that become fully vested, usually after ten to fifteen years of service. Upon retirement, account balances may be used to purchase coverage from a variety of plans offered by the employer or other sources (Shutan, 1999). Pillsbury installed these types of accounts in 1987. Other employers that have used this approach include Chrysler and RJR Nabisco.

Defined Contributions Applied to Medicare

Eli Ginzberg, a well-known health care economist and professor at Columbia University, suggested that Medicare consider shifting away from defined benefits to a defined-contribution approach (stipulating a monetary maximum of governmental outlays) that holds some additional promise of containing the rate of future federal spending (Ginzberg, 1999).

Those who have been wrestling with issues relating to the long-term solvency of the Medicare program talk in terms of "premium support" rather than a defined set of benefits. Writing in the *New England Journal of Medicine,* John Iglehart (1999b, p. 332) says that under such a system, "All beneficiaries would receive a predetermined amount to be applied to the purchase of a health plan providing defined benefits. The amount would vary according to the beneficiary's age, sex, geographic area, health-risk status, income and assets, and use of services." Iglehart adds, "If a beneficiary wanted benefits that went beyond those that could be purchased with the voucher, the amount of which would probably be related to income, he or she would be responsible for the additional cost" (p. 332).

One of the implications of significant numbers of consumers shifting to defined contributions, or premium support, is the likelihood of a dramatic reduction in first-dollar coverage. In other words, by having access to a fixed amount of money, we expect consumers to increase their copayments and deductibles in order to protect themselves against catastrophic health events. Also, by agreeing to pay more up front for a basic benefit package, consumers may be able to expand the scope of their prescription drug coverage and guarantee themselves access to the many expected advances in medical technology described in Chapter Nine.

If this alternative plays out, the ramifications for the U.S. health care system will be profound. Consumers will be in the driver's seat in terms of selecting health plans and dictating the types of coverage they want. Also, one of the drivers of increased health care spending—first-dollar coverage—may of necessity fall out of favor. Managed care plans would have to modify their marketing efforts, focusing more intensely on consumers. And providers would have more difficulty collecting larger deductibles directly from consumers.

Barriers to Defined Contributions

Bruce Vladeck, former HCFA administrator, vigorously disagrees with the notion that premium support for Medicare would save money. Referring to premium support, he says, "It is also a theory with many substantial holes in it, some of which may not be able to be repaired" (Vladeck, 1999, p. 1504). The issues include managing risk selection and adjustment, accounting for cost variations among regions, preventing gaming of the system, and protecting low-income and severely ill beneficiaries.

We also expect that labor unions and some consumer organizations will oppose the growth of defined contributions on the grounds that this model of payment represents an elimination of present medical benefits. In many ways a defined contribution represents a less generous health benefit. But by increasing the predictability of health care spending for employers and HCFA and reducing incentives for inappropriate and unnecessary care, the defined-contribution alternative could represent a significant improvement in the overall cost-effectiveness of the U.S. health care system.

Defined Contributions: Summary

Although defined-contribution models have a long way to go to replace defined benefits, we believe that the payment system is evolving in this direction and that external conditions (such as the expected rapid growth of health care costs for employers and HCFA, consumers' desire for more choice and control, technological advances, and new drugs) will continue to push employers and purchasers toward defined contributions.

Twin Cities Experiment: A Different Model

In 1993 BHCAG rocked the health care industry by issuing a request for proposal (RFP) to a number of health care systems to be the preferred provider for the employees and dependents of twenty-three major Twin Cities employers. BHCAG formed a plan, called Choice Plus, that employees and their families could sign up for; the provider groups would be the health systems selected through the RFP process.

HealthPartners, a large HMO, and HealthSystem Minnesota, an integrated system led by the Park Nicollet Clinic (380 physicians in 1995) and Methodist Hospital (426 beds), were successful bidders. Choice Plus served 90,000 covered lives in the first year, of which 33,500 selected HealthSystem Minnesota as their primary provider (Coddington, Chapman, and Pokoski, 1996).

Buyer's Health Care Action Group Decides to Enhance Consumer Choice

In 1995, for a variety of reasons (including consumers' desire for more freedom of choice and complaints from the health care systems that were not initially selected), BHCAG radically changed its approach. It decided to throw open the doors to all health care systems that could meet its quality and performance criteria. In all, fifteen "care systems" qualified in 1997, the first year (interview with Steve Wetzell, Feb. 12, 1999).

The new Choice Plus plan is sometimes referred to as a "voucher" system. Most BHCAG member companies reimburse employees for the cost of the lowest bidder among the care systems prequalified by BHCAG. As part of this process, care systems submit a budget, which is a combination of unit prices and risk-adjusted estimates of volume of services. Using these cost estimates, BHCAG analyzes the information and creates three cost groups of care systems: low-cost, medium-cost, and high-cost. In the first year Allina, HealthSystem Minnesota, and the Abbott Northwestern Physicians Hospital Organization were the three high-cost care systems.

The care systems ranged from the more advanced integrated systems just mentioned to small groups of primary care physicians who have contractual relationships with specialists and one or more hospitals. Several PHOs were able to meet BHCAG's criteria for inclusion as a care system in the new Choice Plus plan. Medical specialists and hospitals can belong to more than one care system. However, primary care physicians can only belong to a single care system. In 1999 over 95 percent of all primary care physicians in the Twin Cities were participating in one of the BHCAG care systems.

Risk Continues to Reside with Employers

All of the employers are self-insured and responsible for the financial risk. Choice Plus does not reimburse physicians on a capitated basis or otherwise shift insurance risk to providers. Care systems are paid based on the budgets or bids they submit at the beginning of the year, at the usual time when employees select a health plan for the following year.

As noted above, BHCAG has the authority to place a care center in one of the three cost categories. This is important because most employers reimburse employees only for the amount of the low-cost care system; if they elect a higher-cost system, employees pay the difference—about $20 a month in 1997 and 1998 but more in 1999—out of their pockets. This is where similarities with a voucher system come in.

According to Steve Wetzell, executive director of BHCAG:

> Based on what we have observed over the first two years of care systems, there are plenty of incentives for them to retain patients, improve quality and service, and control costs. After each of the first two years, a significant number of employees switched from one of the high-cost care systems (this system also had below average quality and patient satisfaction ratings) to a number of low-cost care systems. Even though we represent a small proportion of employees in the Twin Cities area, and a limited proportion of covered lives for any one care system, these systems take the loss of even a few patients seriously [interview, Feb. 12, 1999].

Choice Plus Increasingly Popular with Employees and Their Families

By late 1999 the number of employers (forty-five) and covered lives (155,000) in Choice Plus had increased substantially from 1994 and 1995, when consumer choice was limited to the two or three health systems selected by BHCAG as part of the RFP process. Employers liked the financial performance of the new system in that annual increases in health care costs were below 5 percent, compared with 10 percent for several of the large HMOs serving the Twin Cities.

Wetzell noted that employees and their families give weight to quality ratings, particularly the results of the patient satisfaction survey. "Rather than selecting a health plan based on informal conversations with neighbors and friends," he told us, "a growing number of employees appear to be approaching this decision more objectively based on data." Wetzell added, "The members of BHCAG have used their market clout to change the fundamentals of the healthcare market in the Twin Cities. That is part of their vision in creating BHCAG; they want to be able to experiment with different approaches to the financing and delivery of healthcare with the hope that the results will be transferable to other parts of the country."

Experts Speak Out on the Buyer's Health Care Action Group Model

John Cochrane, editor of *Integrated Healthcare Report*, refers to the BHCAG model as "a system that rewards value, promotes competition and realigns accountabilities" (1998, p. 9). He goes on to say, "The bottom line for this experiment is that it has restored the consumer to the role of decision-maker and, at the same time, it has made the care systems more competitive and responsive to the consumer. The traditional model for insurance makes the providers more responsive to the health plans" (p. 10). We agree with Cochrane's assessment. He hits on a key theme of this book: providers are becoming more directly responsible to consumers.

Robert Kuttner, author of a number of articles in the *New England Journal of Medicine*, told us that he also is impressed with the BHCAG model. "It measures quality and consumer satisfaction," Kuttner said. "It aligns financial incentives. I think it holds a lot of promise for applications elsewhere."

The concept developed by BHCAG for the Twin Cities market is being tested in other areas of the country. Wetzell noted that the experience in the more rural Sioux Falls, South Dakota, marketplace will be important as a test of the transferability of the Choice Plus model to less populated areas. "We don't see why this model wouldn't work for Medicare, or for any geographic area," he remarked to us. "The main benefit of the Choice Plus model is that it realigns financial incentives. Regardless of the setting, care systems that provide high quality, good service, a broad choice of physicians and hospitals, and low costs, will be rewarded with more patients."

Vouchers and Medical Savings Accounts

There is strong sentiment among a number of health care observers that the employer-based system is crumbling and that it will be replaced by vouchers (another term for defined contributions), MSAs, or some form of individual-insurance model. For example, Roger Battistella and David Burchfield, professors in the Sloan Graduate Program in Health Services Administration at Cornell University, say, "The paternalistic relationship between business and employee health insurance is on its last legs" (Battistella and Burchfield, 1998, p. 24).

Predictions of Increased Use

Battistella and Burchfield (1998, p. 26) state, "Given the financial and regulatory pressures on businesses, the central question is not whether but how employer-sponsored health insurance will change—and what the structure of the new system will be." They consider three alternatives: national health insurance, discontinuation of employee health benefits, and a shift from defined benefits to a defined-contribution strategy. Rejecting the first two, they conclude that "future change predictably will center on medical savings accounts, vouchers or a combination of both" (p. 26).

Vouchers and MSAs have similarities to, and tie in nicely with, defined contributions. However, MSAs and vouchers go further in separating the relationship between employers and employees in terms of control over health benefits.

Medical Savings Accounts

MSAs are available to self-employed individuals, such as sole proprietors and those who earn income from a partnership, limited liability corporation, or S (small business) corporation. If a business has from two to fifty employees, it may set up this type of health plan. MSAs are also available to a limited number of Medicare recipients—390,000 for four years beginning in 1999 (Gemignani, 1997).

The MSA is a combination health plan and tax-free investment plan. Under a pilot program authorized as part of the BBA and limited to 750,000 policyholders, money that a family saves on its insurance premiums by purchasing a high-deductible health policy can be set aside in a specially authorized MSA. Money can be withdrawn from this account at any time, without penalty, to pay medical bills. Of course, consumers have an incentive to let the money remain invested and grow in value on a tax-deferred basis.

MSAs were pioneered by Golden Rule Insurance and have many advocates. However, because of their focus on traditional health plan products, most health insurers do not normally offer these plans. The investment industry does not push MSAs because financial organizations do not normally sell health insurance. Consequently, MSAs have been slow to gain marketplace acceptance.

The possibility of adverse selection—that the healthy would select this type of plan, thus driving up costs for the remaining employees who selected other types of coverage—was an issue when MSAs were first proposed. However, this concern has been largely alleviated by limiting MSAs to the self-employed and to firms employing fewer than fifty workers.

One of the advantages for the self-employed is that they can deduct all of their medical expenses paid out of the MSA. With traditional medical insurance the self-employed can only deduct uncovered medical expenses that exceed 7.5 percent of adjusted gross income and a percentage of health insurance premiums. Most families do not meet this threshold. MSAs place 100 percent of the responsibility back on the individual (Gemignani, 1997). This is why we have grouped MSAs and vouchers together as representing the type of health insurance coverage that puts the consumer in the driver's seat.

The views of Washington, D.C., policy analysts are widely divergent on the future of MSAs. One individual told us, "MSAs are a failed concept; only a few ideologues are holding on." Another individual holds an opposite view: "The limitations placed on MSAs to date almost ensure their failure. They haven't been given a fair trial."

Vouchers and Medical Savings Accounts: Summary

The BHCAG experiment (also referred to as a "voucher approach") and MSAs shift more responsibility for health care decision making to consumers, who have financial incentives to select the highest-quality, most cost-effective provider network. Both vouchers and MSAs represent innovate approaches that deserve to be monitored for what they can teach us that will benefit the public. We believe that both MSAs and vouchers represent an improvement over the present employer-based system with defined benefits.

Individual-Insurance Model

Don Fischer, CEO of the American Medical Group Association, is an advocate of individually owned health insurance. He says, "When you purchase a car, you select the car of your choice and the dealer helps you choose financing that meets your particular needs. Why can't it be the same with healthcare? Your employer doesn't send you to a bank or GMAC and they don't tell you which car you can buy, what color it has to be, and/or where or how fast you can drive it. Healthcare should be no different" (Pricewater-houseCoopers and Lutz, 1999, p. 299).

In 1998 the AMA brought the individual-insurance model back into the limelight after a long absence: "AMA Policy H-165.920 supports individually selected and individually owned health insurance as the preferred method for people to obtain health insurance coverage" (American Medical Association, 1998, p. 1). Exhibit 12.1 is AMA's summary of the advantages of its proposal.

We found many similarities between the AMA proposal and the consumer choice model promoted by the Heritage Foundation a decade ago. Because the AMA model is more recent, we describe it in more detail; however, we also include a summary of main features of the Heritage Foundation proposal in Exhibit 12.2.

Reactions to the Individual-Insurance Model

Following the publication of *The Crisis in Health Care: Costs, Choices, and Strategies* (Coddington, Keen, Moore, and Clarke, 1990), we received a number of opportunities to speak on the subject of the future of the U.S. health care system and how it might be reformed. One of our approaches in these talks was to ask audiences—usually hospital board members, health care executives, physicians, and

Exhibit 12.1. Advantages of the
American Medical Association Proposal.

1. Increases access to adequate health care coverage for all persons, including the self-employed and persons who are disadvantaged economically or by health risk

2. Expands freedom of individuals to choose the source, type, and extent of their health care coverage

3. Increases portability of coverage and job mobility for those in the labor market

4. Reduces the amount of uncompensated or undercompensated care

5. Eliminates inequities in the tax subsidization of insurance spending

6. Reduces incentives to overinsure

7. Provides an opportunity for employers to establish total compensation levels independent of the costs of health care

8. Gives unions the opportunity to assume an expanded role for their members in providing group purchasing mechanisms, education about coverage choices, and negotiation services

9. Offers potential savings to employers in the costs of benefits administration

10. Requires less of a drain on the federal treasury than that which would result from full implementation of present federal legislation and present AMA proposals

11. Enhances use of private sector mechanisms rather than centralized public programs in financing health care

Source: American Medical Association, 1998, p. 2.

employers—which of four health care systems they favored: continuation of the present employer-based system, a modified employer-based system, the single-payer approach, or the consumer choice (individual-insurance) model.

In audience after audience 80 to 90 percent of those present favored the individual-insurance model. Such comments as the following were common:

- "It just makes sense. It would be more like purchasing other types of insurance, like home or automobile coverage."

Exhibit 12.2. Characteristics of the
Heritage Foundation Proposal.

1. Tax credits or vouchers, and deductions; no new taxes. The greater the ratio of health care costs to personal income, the greater the tax benefits.

2. Employers would withhold premiums as they do FICA and state and federal income taxes.

3. Universal coverage is mandated.

4. Employees can maintain their employer-based coverage if they want. However, this would not be their only option.

5. Community rating rather than experience rating (no preexisting conditions disqualify participants or raise premium costs); no cherry picking. Premiums could be varied only on the basis of age, sex, and geography. There could be incentive discounts to promote healthy behavior.

6. Employees could require employers to reimburse them for the cost of health insurance coverage by increasing wages by an equal amount.

7. Portability when employees change jobs or retire.

8. MSAs would be part of this plan.

9. No national health board or government bureaucracies.

Sources: Butler, 1993; Butler and Haislmaier, 1993; Moffit, 1992; Sardegna, 1992; Gavora, 1992.

- "This seems a lot less complex than what we have today, and it has the potential to give us universal coverage to boot."
- "Why isn't there more political support for this type of system? Maybe it's too threatening to the status quo!"
- "This sounds too good to be true! What are the catches? Who pays for it?"

We found the reactions of our audiences surprising (at least at first) and interesting, but we thought that the necessary ingredients for success, such as political support and open and effective information sources, would not facilitate this option. This assessment turned out to be correct; however, this does not mean that individual insurance should not be considered in the future.

Basic Assumption Underlying the American Medical Association Model

One of the basic assumptions embodied in the AMA proposal is that employee fringe benefits, including health insurance, are not a "gift" from employers but are part of the total compensation package. The AMA believes that in a competitive job market, an individual not receiving health insurance should expect to receive a commensurately higher salary.

A second basic feature of the AMA plan is that individuals would receive either federal tax deductions (a subtraction of what is spent on insurance from taxable income) or tax credits (subtraction of the amount spent on insurance from the tax bill). The system would be designed to be revenue neutral for the federal government.

Pluralistic Emphasis

The AMA proposal does not mandate that employers stop providing health benefits. Rather, it offers an alternative to employers. "It allows for a natural evolution to a system where all health expense coverage may become individually owned to the extent that individual choices over time dictate it" (American Medical Association, 1998, p. 4).

Tax Treatment

The AMA proposal suggests tax credits for a predetermined portion of the cost of individually owned health plan coverage. This would encourage those who are uninsured to get coverage; the net cost for those in the lower income brackets would be zero. "Persons whose incomes are too low to have an income tax liability could still purchase coverage and file to receive a refundable credit that would be directly paid to them" (American Medical Association, 1998, p. 6).

One of the frequent questions about the individually owned health insurance model is how to make sure that the uninsured purchase coverage. As noted in Chapter Eleven, a significant number of the uninsured have access to health insurance coverage from employers but are unwilling to pay their share of the premium; therefore they decline the coverage.

Robert Moffit, who is on the staff of the Heritage Foundation, describes how the tax system would be used to encourage coverage for all Americans: "Under the Heritage proposal [which is similar to the AMA plan] every American family, regardless of employment status, would receive a voucher or tax credit in place the current tax exclusion [for those who receive health benefits through their employer]. Families could use that tax relief for health insurance, out-of-pocket medical costs, or a tax-free medical savings account from which they could pay medical bills directly. The tax relief would be targeted at need. Using a sliding scale of refundable tax credits, more help would go to families with low incomes or high medical bills" (Arnett, 1999, p. 48). Moffit adds, "As a condition for receiving a credit or voucher, the head of every family would be required to purchase at least a basic package of catastrophic coverage" (p. 48). He notes that an econometric analysis showed that virtually every income group in the United States would be better off under a tax credit system, with families earning $30,000 to $40,000 a year benefiting the most.

Purchasing Cooperatives

The AMA advocates the formation of group purchasing cooperatives by groups other than employers, with emphasis on the formation of national or regional pools. The rationale for the national and regional scope recommendation is to provide a choice of plans and to facilitate portability of coverage for those changing jobs (American Medical Association, 1998). As noted earlier in this chapter, some human resources representatives believe that this will be time consuming and difficult.

The AMA refers to purchasing organizations as "voluntary choice cooperatives" (VCCs). Nancy Dickey and Peter McMenamin of the AMA say, "Choosing a health plan through a VCC would be a new experience for many patients, but analogous systems, such as the Federal Employees Health Benefits Program, have shown that this approach can be successful" (Dickey and McMenamin, 1999, p. 1305).

Risk Adjustment

Under this proposal risk adjustments would be used in determining the amount of an employer's direct contributions toward individually purchased coverage (American Medical Association, 1998). Without risk adjustment some employers would end up paying substantially more than they do today, and there would be no financial incentive to change to the individually purchased plans.

The AMA proposal differs on this point from the consumer choice model proposed by the Heritage Foundation. The Heritage Foundation would use community rating with risk adjustments for age and sex only, whereas the AMA proposal would leave experience rating intact for fear of the negative impact of community rating on employers with large numbers of younger and healthier workers.

Financial Models: Providers' Perspective

This chapter has described payment system models from the perspective of the employer, Medicare and Medicaid, and the consumer. What about physicians, hospitals, long-term care providers, drug manufacturers, and others who provide health care products and services? What will the payment system of the future look like from their perspective?

A few years ago we would have agreed that global capitation—physicians and hospitals paid a single PMPM rate—would have become the dominant payment methodology of the new millennium. However, it has not worked out that way.

Myth: Capitation Is Growing

Jeffrey Barbakow, CEO of Tenet, believes that "anticipating the clinical needs and utilization patterns for entire populations, and pricing them appropriately, will be central to the future economic viability of the hospital industry" (Gilkey, 1999, p. 99). This sounds like a vision of the future involving more capitated payment.

James Robinson, professor of health economics at the University of California-Berkeley, talks about the "recent rapid spread of capitation contracting and delegation of utilization management. Large provider organizations have begun to contract with health plans on a capitated basis for primary, specialty, and, increasingly, hospital and pharmacy services" (Robinson, 1999, p. 11).

In our view the conclusion of Barbakow and Robinson that capitation is gaining in popularity reflects the perspective of those who focus on a limited number of more advanced managed care markets. On the contrary, we see no evidence that capitation is increasing in most parts of the country. In fact, capitation appears to be falling out of favor with many health plans and provider groups. This finding was confirmed in our focus group discussion with the chief financial officers of eight large health care systems representing over two hundred hospitals and thousands of physicians.

On a more quantitative basis an AMA study showed that the proportion of physician practice revenues from capitated contracts fell from 8.4 percent in 1996 to 7 percent in 1997. The same research showed that in 1997, 80 percent of HMOs reimbursed physicians on a fee-for-service basis, up from 74.9 percent in 1996 ("1999 Industry Outlook," 1999).

Mix of Discounted Fee-for-Service and Capitation More Likely

Robert Mittman of the Institute for the Future offers these observations about capitated payment versus a mixed system of reimbursement: "To read the healthcare press and seminar announcements, one would gather that capitation has taken the health industry by storm. In fact, despite years of growth, capitation has reached only 10 percent of physician reimbursement. And global capitation—the type that makes a real difference in provider behavior—accounts for only four percent of physician payment in the U.S. A provider organization that retooled itself for full, global capitation next year would be making a strategic mistake" (Institute for the Future, 1999, p. 2). Mittman says that health care organizations that fail to prepare for the complex and mixed reimbursement forms that are likely to continue to emerge in the next several years would also be making a mistake. We agree.

What Is Stopping Capitation?

Why has capitation failed to become the payment system of choice? Table 12.1 presents our assessment of the pros and cons of capitation. The negatives appear to outweigh the positives.

Table 12.1. Pros and Cons of Global Capitation.

Pros	Cons
Makes medical costs more predictable for health plans and employers	Insufficient number of medical groups capable of performing medical management and accepting risk
Aligns financial incentives among health plans, physicians, and hospitals	Size of many markets too small for reasonable number of covered lives
Promotes investment in clinical guidelines and other quality initiatives	Health plans' resistance to dismantling internal medical management and actuarial capabilities
Should save money for health plans, employers, governmental payers, and consumers	Health plans do not want to give away potential windfall profits associated with drop in inpatient utilization
	Puts too much power in the hands of PCPs at the expense of specialists and hospitals
	More difficult to administer than fee-for-service
	Consumers resist loss of freedom of choice that goes with global capitation

As Table 12.1 suggests, capitation works best where there is a large population base and a significant surplus of physicians, criteria met by Southern California and a few other densely populated areas but not by most other parts of the country. It is extremely difficult to capitate physicians, medical groups, and hospitals in sparsely populated areas. Statistical analysis and probability theory do not work as well in these kinds of situations, and physicians are unlikely to be motivated to participate. One of the authors remembers interviewing thirty physicians in small towns in northwestern Kansas about their willingness to participate in capitated contracting. It was not a pleasant experience!

Second, many would argue that a primary factor holding back the growth of capitation is the lack of a sufficient number of large and well-organized medical groups. It is difficult to develop capitation models that work in an IPA or loosely knit PHO; the decision making and financial self-interests of potential participants are nearly impossible to align. There are not enough tightly organized multispecialty groups with significant market presence to cover most of the country. And even if the consolidation of physician practices continues, the pace is not fast enough to yield a significant number of large multispecialty groups that are well suited to provide health care on a globally capitated basis.

Finally, not all health plans are interested in globally capitating physicians and hospitals. They are well aware of the immediate reductions in inpatient utilization and visits to specialists that will result, and the health plans want to keep these savings, not pass windfall profits on to providers.

Fee-for-Service Plans Are Not the Answer

At the same time, discounted fee-for-service payment has not solved the problem of inappropriate utilization. The lower the payment rates per diagnosis or procedure, the greater the number of procedures. Roger Gilbertson, CEO of MeritCare (a physician-led integrated system) in Fargo, North Dakota, told us, "You decrease unit prices, and you are going to increase utilization." There is plenty of evidence supporting the view that this is the way things work in health care.

Columbine Example

PacifiCare found this to be true in paying specialists who were part of the Columbine Medical Group, an IPA that until 1999 exclusively served all four hundred thousand of PacifiCare's covered lives in the Denver area. With a stable base of subscribers and no significant changes in reimbursement levels, medical specialists in Columbine registered an 81 percent increase in the number of procedures performed on PacifiCare's covered lives over the period from 1995 through 1998. During the same four-year period PCPs, who were capitated, registered a 21 percent increase in the number of visits, tests, and procedures.

John Gates (1999), former CEO of Columbine and founder of Millennial Healthcare, said that physicians on the Columbine board told him that the growth was due to patient demands and the availability of technology. We suspect that there is another factor at work: the desire on the part of many specialists to maintain or increase their revenues.

Piecework

James Reinertsen, former CEO of HealthSystem Minnesota, believes the piecework fostered by fee-for-service payment is a huge barrier to innovation in health care. "Piecework," he says, "has been found to be a serious problem in almost every other industry, where it has largely been eliminated. The healthcare industry is one of the few places where it still persists. And it is a major system barrier to clinical improvement" (1994, p. 23).

What Is the Answer?

We conclude that efforts to shift the risk to physicians and hospitals—such as capitated payment—are unlikely to grow in importance in most parts of the United States. Health plans are more likely to control utilization, or volume of specialist and hospital visits, using their increasingly sophisticated information systems and databases combined with financial incentives. Even large employers that contract directly with providers on behalf of their employees are developing the tools to control utilization.

HCFA has been relying on DRGs to control inpatient costs and is moving to a similar model for outpatient services. These approaches, combined with increasingly sophisticated information systems, should allow Medicare to better control inappropriate utilization of hospital inpatient and outpatient services.

The larger integrated systems that effectively combine physician organizations and hospitals continue to invest in clinical guidelines to reduce clinical variation, and this should help control inappropriate health care costs.

Conclusions

We believe that most of the payment system models described in this chapter represent improvements over both the present employer-based system and direct payment of providers by HCFA. Each one would speed up the process of shifting more responsibility to consumers for their own health care. The role of the middleman—employers—would be reduced. From a physician and hospital perspective, we do not expect that the changes on the horizon will translate into increased use of capitated payment for physicians and hospitals.

Part Four combines the payment system models with a number of the external factors covered in Part Three (such as consumerism, technology, consolidation, and federal policy initiatives) and with economic conditions in order to identify and describe four scenarios for the future. This is followed by an assessment of the four scenarios in terms of which one best serves the public interest and which is most likely to come to pass during the first five years of the twenty-first century.

Part Four

Beyond Managed Care
Scenarios for the Future

*America seems to be committed to a particular path—
seeking cost control through managed care, increasingly
using shareholder-owned HMOs, and relying heavily on
financial incentives for physicians. Though innovation
is possible along this broad path, other, potentially
superior paths are precluded.*
ROBERT KUTTNER, "Must Good HMOs Go Bad?
The Search for Checks and Balances," *New England
Journal of Medicine*, 1998

The two chapters in Part Four present our analysis of where health care may be headed in the future. The first analysis is more idealistic and hopeful; the second is more practical.

Chapter Thirteen combines the various payment system models reviewed in Chapter Twelve with a number of additional factors likely to shape health care in the future (see Figure P.2).

In Chapter Fourteen we analyze each scenario, using ten criteria that represent what we would consider the best health care system for the United States. We also assess the probability that each scenario will come into being in the first five years of the new millennium.

Figure P.2. Four Scenarios and the Factors
Likely to Shape Health Care, 2000–2005.

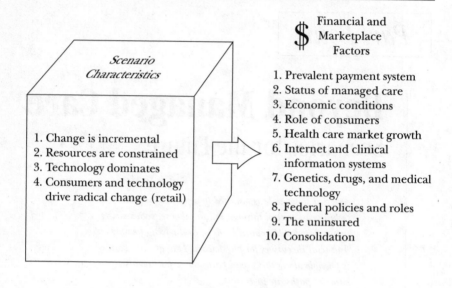

Scenario Characteristics

1. Change is incremental
2. Resources are constrained
3. Technology dominates
4. Consumers and technology drive radical change (retail)

$ Financial and Marketplace Factors

1. Prevalent payment system
2. Status of managed care
3. Economic conditions
4. Role of consumers
5. Health care market growth
6. Internet and clinical information systems
7. Genetics, drugs, and medical technology
8. Federal policies and roles
9. The uninsured
10. Consolidation

Four Health Care Scenarios

> *I have been in this business for close to thirty years,*
> *but I have never been so confused over where health care*
> *is headed. I know this: the present system in not*
> *sustainable. But what will take its place?*
>
> HEALTH SYSTEM CEO

In this chapter we propose four scenarios depicting the possible shape of health care over the first five years of the new century:

1. Incremental change
2. Resources constrained
3. Technology dominates
4. Consumerism and technology (retail)

The four scenarios are not mutually exclusive. For example, the trend toward consumerism in health care would grow in any of the scenarios. However, scenario 4 would represent the most extreme case, including significant changes in payment system models that demand greater consumer involvement, decision making, and financial participation. The development and use of technology is another theme that runs through all scenarios; however, in scenarios 3 and 4 technological change would be the most advanced.

In reviewing the four scenarios, one physician-administrator remarked, "I don't think that any of the four scenarios would come into being just as you have posed them. However, I believe that the future would contain elements of all of the scenarios." We agree with this assessment. Our main purpose in presenting the scenarios is to challenge thinking about the future in terms of how the forces we have discussed in this book are likely to play out during the first five years of the new millennium.

We have not included the changing demographics of Americans, mainly the aging of the population and the growth in the Hispanic and other minority communities, as a variable among the four scenarios considered in this chapter. The aging of the population will happen regardless of which of the scenarios is dominant—it is a given. The growing number of frail elderly will consume an increasing share of health care resources.

Scenario 1: Incremental Change

In this scenario we view managed care as a mature industry. The trends of the late 1990s identified in earlier chapters would continue, but these would not represent anything remotely resembling a fundamental market shift. The characteristics of scenario 1 are summarized in Exhibit 13.1.

During the next five years there would be conferences for physicians on topics such as how to keep managed care from driving you out of business, using clinical information to improve quality and financial results, and how to avoid being treated like a commodity. Issues facing hospitals would revolve around performance improvement, coping with the BBA, and improving the financial performance of hospital-owned medical practices. An increasingly popular subject would be learning how to market directly to consumers and the self-pay markets.

Prevalent Payment System

The incremental-change scenario includes elements of three of the payment system models discussed in Chapter Twelve: slow growth in commercial managed care, limited growth in Medicare+ Choice, and some increase in the corporate use of defined contributions in place of defined benefits.

In this scenario employer-based health care would continue to be the most common source of coverage for employees and their families. However, an increasing proportion of employers (close to

Exhibit 13.1. Characteristics of Scenario 1: Incremental Change.

Financial and Marketplace Factors	*Characteristics*
1. Prevalent payment system	1. Employer-based system with continued movement toward defined contributions
2. Status of managed care	2. Growth opportunities in Medicare; commercial managed care is a mature market; emphasis on how to make managed care work better
3. Economic conditions	3. Continuation of strong economy and growing equity markets
4. Role of consumers	4. Role of consumers continues to grow but is not dominant
5. Health care market growth	5. $1.8 trillion by 2005; continued movement into private-pay market niches
6. Internet and clinical information systems	6. Internet use increases dramatically but progress in clinical information systems is slow
7. Genetics, drugs, and medical technology	7. Rapid growth expected but with major issues revolving around payment for new drugs and advanced technology
8. Federal policies	8. Federal policy focuses on making managed care more consumer friendly (for example, patients' bill of rights, mandated coverages)
9. The uninsured	9. Reach 55 million by 2005
10. Consolidation	10. Hospital and medical group consolidation continue but at a slow pace

half) would have at least partially converted to cafeteria plans or defined contributions. This means that employees and their families would be making more of the decisions on the type of health plan coverage they want (for example, analyzing the trade-offs between higher copayments and deductibles and better drug and catastrophic coverage).

Status of Managed Care

Under scenario 1 managed care would continue to grow but at a much slower pace than in previous years. Health plan consolidation would continue, with two or three large health plans dominating most metropolitan areas. Discounted fee-for-service payment would continue to be the most common way of paying physicians. Capitated payment of physicians would not gain ground or become the norm.

In this scenario we anticipate minor modifications in the BBA that would make Medicare HMOs and other managed care initiatives more attractive to providers and beneficiaries and take some financial pressures off hospitals. However, this scenario anticipates limited growth in Medicare managed care—to between 30 and 35 percent of the eligible population by 2005 (compared with just over 15 percent in 2000).

We expect managed care plans to be available to 95 percent of all employees of firms offering health insurance coverage (compared with 85 percent in 2000). Total HMO enrollment, including Medicare and Medicaid, would approach one hundred million, or one-third of all Americans. Again, scenario 1 is a picture of managed care as a mature industry, and with the exception of Medicare, an industry with limited growth potential.

Economic Conditions

This scenario anticipates a continuing strong U.S. economy, little inflation, and no major discontinuities in the equity markets. Unemployment would remain low, and corporate earnings and employment would remain relatively high.

The wealth accumulated by many Americans by virtue of their investments in the stock market and in their retirement programs may not grow as rapidly as over the past five years. Real income levels would increase, and more Americans should have significant financial resources to spend on discretionary medical services.

Role of Consumers

One of the themes of this book is the trend toward greater consumer decision making and power, and this would continue under the incremental-change scenario. The number of radio, television, newspaper, magazine, and billboard advertisements for health care products would exceed those of the late 1990s.

We would expect double-digit growth in the purchase and use of CAM and increased coverage of CAM by health plans. As part of this, traditional physicians would increasingly accept these alternative "nonscientific" approaches, incorporate CAM into their practices, and be more willing to work with consumers in meeting their total health care needs.

Consumers would become increasingly demanding of health care providers, hospitals, and health plans. The pressure would be on providers to offer significantly more value (for example, higher quality, better service, convenience, innovation). Even under the incremental-change scenario, providers would have their hands full meeting growing consumer expectations, much of it driven by advertising.

Health Care Market Growth

In the incremental-change scenario, the health care market would increase from $1.3 trillion in 2000 to $1.8 trillion in 2005. Hospitals would provide more intensive care and generate more revenues, but the long-term trend of hospitals' declining share of total health care spending would continue. Hospitals would experience greater problems in hiring and retaining health care professionals and support staff.

Physicians and medical groups would maintain their 20 percent share of the market, and dental and vision services as a proportion of the total would be unlikely to change much. However, drugs, medical equipment, long-term care, rehabilitation, home health, and other personal and medical services would increase in relative importance.

Internet and Clinical Information Systems

Many aspects of the Internet and IT advances already affecting health care would grow in importance. This includes consumer use of the Internet for medical information and support groups and use of e-mail between physicians and patients.

We expect that many medical groups, hospital systems, and integrated health care organizations would increase their investment in clinical IT, including EMRs and longitudinal databases. But within the five-year time frame used in this analysis, the results would be of marginal value for most organizations. However, consumers would take to the computerized records and increasingly demand that providers use this type of technology. At the same time we expect growth in independent companies that provide EMR services for consumers.

Large health plans would have increasingly sophisticated databases originating from their claims payment records. These databases would be used to identify top-performing physicians and medical groups and to root out doctors whose performance is marginal.

Genetics, Drugs, and Medical Technology

On the prescription drug side we anticipate a growing number of new drugs, many targeted toward chronic and other common (and high volume) diseases. Many of these drugs would have been enhanced as a result of genetic research, and they would be expensive. The flow of advanced medical diagnostic and treatment devices would exceed that experienced over the past five years.

We expect a number of employer-sponsored health plans to expand their drug benefits. Most consumers, including those on Medicare, would either purchase supplemental policies that provide outpatient drug coverage or pay for drugs out of their pockets.

Federal Policies

We expect Congress and the executive branch to give limited financial relief to hospitals by relaxing some of the more onerous provisions of the BBA. It is unlikely that Medicare payments to physicians and hospitals would return to the levels of their heyday, but reimbursement levels should be better than originally specified in the BBA. In order to boost Medicare+Choice HCFA is also likely to find ways to make payment to managed care organizations more attractive.

Passage of a patient's bill of rights, mandating more benefits, and other legislation requiring certain HMO practices (such as longer lengths of stay for maternity cases) would be a primary concern of Congress, the executive branch, and many states. This would be accompanied by added costs; therefore HMOs would be less competitive with PPOs. Of course, HMOs would continue to fight back with expanded information on clinical outcomes and other measures of the health status of members. It would be a battle of those with quantitative data on health status, patient satisfaction, and clinical outcomes versus those relying on anecdotal evidence.

We anticipate that medical groups and physician networks (including PHOs and IPAs) would face continuing challenges related to the pricing of services and other perceived anticompetitive practices. In other words the Federal Trade Commission and Justice Department would be actively seeking out physicians and medical groups they believe are colluding in pricing their services.

The Uninsured

Under the incremental-change scenario, we expect the number of the uninsured to reach fifty-five million by 2005, or 18 percent of the population (compared with 16 percent in 2000). This increase, combined with a tightening of Medicare payment levels, would contribute to increasingly serious financial problems for many hospitals and health systems.

Consolidation

The most noticeable consolidation would be among health plans; start-up HMOs would find it even more difficult to succeed than in the 1990s. But contrary to conventional wisdom, we do not expect to see the disappearance of provider-owned health plans that focus on local markets.

For the first two years of the new millennium, health plans would attempt to use their market power to reduce medical loss ratios and spread overhead over a larger base, thus improving profit margins. We expect health plans to be only marginally successful in this strategy. As noted earlier, health plans would also push for higher premiums, but we expect more resistance from employers than in 1998 and 1999.

Physicians would continue to consolidate into larger groups, but the process would be slow and steady, not spectacular. We do not anticipate a resurgence of the growth of the PPM industry and its efforts to consolidate medical groups. At the same time medical groups that are aggressive, long-term investors need capital partners; such medical groups would therefore combine with other medical groups or with hospitals.

Hospital consolidation would continue under this scenario but at a moderate pace. Because we do not expect the BBA to be as limiting as in its 1999 form, we do not anticipate wholesale closures of hospitals, even in inner-city or rural areas.

Scenario 1: Summary

This scenario assumes that the emerging trends of the late 1990s will continue into the first five years of the new century. In a sense the health care future under the incremental-change scenario is fairly predictable. It is not an altogether unpleasant view of the future, at least for physicians, hospitals, and drug manufacturers. However, it would be unattractive for the uninsured, employers offering health benefits, and HCFA.

Scenario 2: Constrained Resources

Under this scenario (summarized in Exhibit 13.2) health care would face serious cutbacks in payment levels and would experience instability. Driven by uncertain and generally poor economic conditions, employers and HCFA would be under increasing pressure to control costs. Those segments of health care most dependent on consumers' discretionary spending would be in for difficult times. Medicare's financial problems would be greater than anticipated in the 1999 planning effort by Congress and

HCFA staff, and the pressures to reduce payments to providers would accelerate.

In the 1990s many hospitals and health plans lost money on operations but made it up in the extremely robust performance of their financial investments. The chief financial officer of a large multihospital system told us that revenues from operations were not covering costs in the late 1990s; this pattern would become more prevalent in this scenario.

Regarding earnings from investments, it was reported that all BCBS plans combined earned net income of $1.4 billion in 1998.

Exhibit 13.2. Characteristics of Scenario 2:
Constrained Resources.

Financial and Marketplace Factors	*Characteristics*
1. Prevalent payment system	1. Employer-based system moves more rapidly into defined contributions and vouchers
2. Status of managed care	2. Traditional HMO plans grow more rapidly than PPOs
3. Economic conditions	3. Economic uncertainty, a recessionary period, and at least one significant stock market decline
4. Role of consumers	4. Required to pay a bigger share of premiums and higher copayments and deductibles; less discretionary spending on health-related services
5. Health care market growth	5. $1.6 to $1.7 trillion by 2005
6. Internet and clinical information systems	6. Investment in clinical information systems declines; Internet use levels off
7. Genetics, drugs, and medical technology	7. Demand is weaker than in other scenarios, and sales of new drugs and technology slow
8. Federal policies	8. HCFA takes a tough stance toward health plans, physicians, and hospitals
9. The uninsured	9. Reach record levels—60 to 65 million
10. Consolidation	10. Health plan, physician, and hospital consolidation increase

As Martin Weiss, chairman of a bond-rating agency, attests, "The stock market has been a life-saver for many of these companies. What remains to be seen is how they will fare if the stock market does not continue to rise" (Rauber, 1999, p. 14). This situation is portrayed in the cartoon shown as Figure 13.1.

Health care conferences and conventions would be less well attended than in the past, with more interest in audio- and video-conferencing to save travel expenses. Popular topics for hospital administrators might include balancing declining revenues with community needs, collaboration to cut costs, and learning to live with less. Physicians would be bombarded with opportunities to attend meetings dealing with survival strategies in a down market, evaluating whether it is time to consolidate, and adjusting income expectations for the future.

Prevalent Payment System

In this scenario the emphasis would be on moving more employees and Medicare recipients into defined contribution models, MSAs, vouchers, and similar arrangements that limit employer spending. HCFA would be under pressure to increase its use of

Figure 13.1.

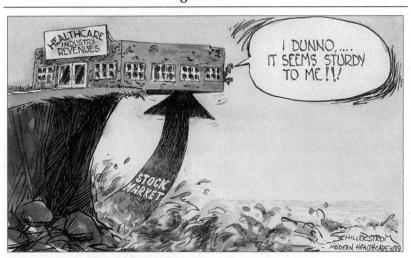

Source: Modern Healthcare; used with the permission of Roger Schillerstrom.

HMOs and PSOs, and the percentage of Medicare recipients in HMOs would approach 50 percent.

Status of Managed Care

As it became obvious that PPOs had failed in their efforts to control costs for employers, traditional HMOs would grow faster than in scenario 1. HMOs would be partially successful in improving their earnings by reducing the medical loss ratio (for example, through lower payments to physicians and hospitals and limiting payment for most name brand drugs) and reducing their marketing and overhead expenses. They would not be successful in increasing premiums enough to cover significantly higher medical costs.

The trend of slower growth in the number of HMO covered lives would reverse, and the proportion of employees and families eligible for PPO services would decline. Employers would offer employees fewer alternatives, and cost-effectiveness would be the major factor in deciding which health plans would be retained. By taking business from PPOs, HMOs would begin to grow rapidly, no longer appearing to be a mature industry.

Economic Conditions

Those who assign the highest probability to this scenario believe that the favorable economic conditions of the 1990s cannot continue for another five years. The economy of the 1990s has been called the "Goldilocks" economy—neither too hot (requiring increased interest rates) nor too cold. As one article warns, "Americans like happy endings. Unfortunately, they seem to have forgotten the conclusion of the Goldilocks story: the bears chased her away" ("Goldilocks or Gridlock?", 1999, p. 17).

We are not forecasting a depression. Rather, this scenario would include a two-year period of economic uncertainty and at least one decline serious enough to qualify as a recession (three consecutive quarters of negative growth in the GDP). Unemployment would increase but not reach 10 percent of the workforce. Home prices in many markets would fall, and overall inflation would be near zero; but the situation would not be serious enough to trigger the kind of worldwide deflationary spiral sometimes predicted in 1999.

Business earnings would decline, and the prospect of this reduction in profits would precipitate at least one long-term decline (of at least 20 percent) in the Dow Jones Industrial Average. The high-tech stocks dominating the Nasdaq would be down even more. The net worth of many retirees and others with large retirement and profit-sharing portfolios would drop in value. Psychologically, many people would feel poorer than during the late 1990s.

Role of Employers

Employers, under pressure to maintain earnings, would increasingly turn to defined contributions for their employee health care benefits. A number of organizations would drop health care coverage altogether. Managers and unions would more frequently clash on the issue of health benefits. There would be heightened interest in exploring the value of an individual insurance payment system. Some "radicals" would begin advocating a Canadian-style single-payer model.

Role of Consumers

Despite more restrictive health plan alternatives, consumers would find ways to play a bigger role. Under this scenario consumers would lose some of the freedom of choice that has been building in the 1990s with the growth of PPOs and POS HMOs. The options provided by employers would be more restrictive, and consumers would be asked to pay a larger portion in premiums, copayments, and deductibles. In many respects this would represent a continuation of the trend of the late 1990s but at an accelerated pace.

At the same time consumers would become more self-reliant. This would mean greater use of the Internet for health information and support groups, increased reliance on alternative medicines and wellness, more self-care, and more attention to the costs of various health care treatment alternatives. There would be greater acceptance of telephone triage and the use of physician's assistants and nurse practitioners. Under the constrained-resources scenario a large number of consumers would cut back on their discretionary spending for laser eye surgery, face-lifts, and lifestyle drugs.

Health Care Market Growth

Health care expenditures would not reach the levels forecast in the incremental-change scenario ($1.8 trillion by 2005). Instead, health care spending would be in the range of $1.6 to $1.7 trillion. Falling short of the spending projected under scenario 1 would be the direct result of employers and HCFA taking stronger stands on controlling health care costs and consumers reducing their discretionary health-related spending.

Internet and Clinical Information Systems

Consumers' use of the Internet would level off under this scenario. However, investment by medical groups and hospitals in clinical information systems would decline, and the widespread application of these new systems, and the expected benefits, would be delayed.

Genetics, Drugs, and Medical Technology

Under tighter economic conditions leading to increased efforts to reduce health care costs, as well as continuing pressure from Medicare, spending on new drugs and medical technology would drop below the levels anticipated under the incremental-change scenario. These two categories would still grow rapidly, at the expense of physicians and hospitals, but more slowly than the pharmaceutical and high-tech companies had planned. Research and development spending by pharmaceutical companies would be at lower levels than in the incremental-change scenario.

Federal Policies

It is doubtful that there would be large federal budget surpluses available to bail out Medicare. New studies would show that the Medicare system is likely to reach insolvency earlier than previously forecast. Therefore the pressure would be on for Congress and the administration to find new ways to limit Medicare spending. Drugs for outpatient use would have little chance of being added to the Medicare benefits package unless this added benefit also contained consumer payment provisions and a means test.

Despite the recommendations of MedPAC, Medicare reimbursement for hospitals would not be adequate to cover full overhead allocations. HCFA would increasingly buy hospital services on the basis of short-term marginal costs. As a result, the number of failures or mergers of inner-city and rural hospitals would double over what could be expected in the incremental-change scenario.

Efforts designed to achieve full compliance with federal regulations on reimbursement of medical groups and hospitals would be vigorously enforced. Consequently, providers would increase their diligence in implementing corporate compliance programs. We would hear many more comments like that of the neurosurgeon who said, "I feel like we have a spy in our midst."

The Uninsured

Under the less favorable economic conditions that are part of this scenario, and absent any new federal programs, the ranks of the uninsured would reach sixty to sixty-five million, or 20 to 22 percent of the population. This increase in the uninsured population would be driven by a number of medium-sized employers dropping health benefits, by higher costs to employees, and by the higher unemployment rate. This compares with fifty-five million uninsured in 2005 in the incremental-change scenario and would represent a serious destabilizing factor for health care.

Consolidation

Many small health plans would fail, and those with the deepest pockets—the large national insurance companies—would continue to gain market power. Many physician groups and hospitals would give up on their health plans, and others that had been considering the formation of their own HMO or PSO would table these plans.

Hospital consolidation and collaboration, especially among not-for-profit community hospitals, would accelerate. Hospital board members would become increasingly nervous about the future of their organizations, especially in light of tighter HCFA payment schedules and the consolidation of managed care plans. Investor-owned hospital systems would have difficulty demonstrating earnings growth, and the value of the stock of these companies would drop, making new acquisitions prohibitively expensive.

Physicians and medical groups would find themselves in a quandary. Many solo practitioners and small single-specialty groups would hunker down, keep their fixed costs (including physician salaries) as low as possible, and attempt to ride out the economic storm and the desire of payers to cut health care costs. Other physicians would join larger groups as a way of gaining financial stability. The problem, however, is that most medical groups do not have significant financial reserves; consequently, physicians would have to take pay cuts if their practices were to survive. Interest among physicians in joining unions would be the highest of any of the scenarios. An increasing number of specialists, especially in metropolitan areas where there are substantial surpluses, would be driven out of business or forced to relocate.

Scenario 2: Summary

The *Wall Street Journal* basically summarized the constrained-resources scenario: "When the next economic downturn hits, many employers and individuals will dump their costly medical coverage, throwing more people into the ranks of the uninsured and renewing calls for government intervention. Unless the industry figures out how to re-engineer healthcare to improve both quality and efficiency, it could even be replaced by a government system" (Rundle, 1999, p. A1).

Physicians' complaints about managed care in the 1990s would seem trivial compared with the stress on health care providers resulting from concerted efforts to cut health care costs and generally weak economic conditions. The pressures on hospitals, especially those that are small, undercapitalized, or in rural areas, would be untenable. Any residual Wall Street interest in health care would all but disappear.

Scenario 3: Technology Dominant

Under the technology-dominant scenario (summarized in Exhibit 13.3), the development and application of technology would far exceed the expectations of the late 1990s. The prediction Bill Gates (1999, p. xxii) made would come to pass: "The successful companies of the next decade will be the ones that use digital tools to reinvent the way they work. These companies will make decisions quickly, act efficiently, and directly touch their customers in positive ways."

Exhibit 13.3. Characteristics of Scenario 3: Technology Dominant.

Financial and Marketplace Factors	Characteristics
1. Prevalent payment system	1. Defined contributions, vouchers, MSAs
2. Status of managed care	2. Unable to control costs for employers; more consolidation
3. Economic conditions	3. Strong worldwide and U.S. economy
4. Role of consumers	4. Consumers have the financial clout and responsibility to make more of their own health care decisions
5. Health care market growth	5. $1.9 trillion by 2005
6. Internet and clinical information systems	6. Consumers demand more sophisticated information systems and use Internet extensively
7. Genetics, drugs, and medical technology	7. Many consumers able to afford new drugs and technology; health plans find ways to offer new products that include new drugs
8. Federal policies	8. Funding for Medicare highest of any of the scenarios
9. The uninsured	9. Drop somewhat from previous scenarios but still are in the 30 to 35 million range
10. Consolidation	10. Pressures for health plan consolidation but not so much for physicians and hospitals

Here is a sampling of what might be expected in terms of the development and application of technology:

- *Internet.* By 2005 nearly every home would have Internet access via high-speed transmission. Although the number of health-related Web sites would increase, a handful of highly credible sites would dominate. Most medical groups of five or more physicians would have their own Web sites, and this would be linked to other clinic Web sites. Consumer e-mail communication with physicians would be commonplace.

- *Telehealth.* The potential for telehealth dreamed about in the late 1990s would become a reality by 2005. Monitoring of patients in their homes would be routine, thus reducing the need for home health visits.

- *Information systems.* Referring primarily to clinical and enterprise-wide information systems, the development of these systems would accelerate, and at least half of all hospitals and most large medical groups would have fully developed EMRs. At the same time many consumers would assume ownership of their medical records, and new ventures offering medical record services directly to consumers would be common. Many integrated systems, hospitals, and larger medical groups would be far along in developing a "digital nervous system" that provides real-time information for both clinical and management decision making.

- *Genetic research.* With the Human Genome Project completed ahead of schedule, the value of the findings would surprise the skeptics. Gene therapy would advance faster than expected. The knowledge base available for developing new drugs would exceed the expectations of all but a few visionary leaders.

- *New drugs.* The number of new drugs put on the market would exceed the pace of introduction of drugs in the late 1990s by a factor of two to three times. Furthermore, claims by drug companies that these new therapies would reduce many types of surgical interventions and inpatient days in hospitals would prove to be correct. Advances in medications would reduce the need for some types of surgery (for example, open-heart surgery).

- *Advances in medical technology.* There would be at least two major breakthroughs the equivalent of laparoscopic surgery and the MRI and hundreds of smaller advances affecting every medical specialty. (Chapter Nine included examples of several of these incremental technological advances.) The net effect: medicine as it was known in the late 1990s would be radically changed. Physicians unable to invest in the new technologies or unwilling to be trained to use them and incorporate them into their practices would be hard pressed to stay in business. The pressures on hospitals to purchase new technology would be greater than ever, and the gap between the kinds of services offered by inner-city and rural hospitals on the one hand and tertiary care and academic centers on the other would grow.

The combination of all of these factors would lead to a health care system far different from the one existing at the turn of the century. In many respects the availability of technology would proceed more rapidly than the payment mechanisms; this would lead to a number of issues for HCFA, health plans, and providers.

The best-attended professional seminars and conferences would include topics like technology and strategy, new business models for a technological age, and paying for all the things that can be done. Physicians would attend conferences on subjects like working in partnership with well-educated consumers and the uses and abuses of clinical outcomes data.

Prevalent Payment System

As discussed in Chapter Four, technology has been a major driver of past increases in health care spending. Because of the dominance of technological advances in this scenario, health care costs for payers would be the highest of any of the four scenarios.

One of the struggles of this scenario would be to modify payment system models to keep pace with the development and application of technology. For example, how should physicians be compensated for consulting with patients about information pulled from Web sites or for consultations via telemedicine? Would the health plans be able to come up with new insurance products that include access to new drugs and medical technology? Would compensation be tied to risk-adjusted medical outcomes?

Because their health benefit costs would be increasing more rapidly than expected, employers would move aggressively toward use of defined contributions, vouchers, and MSAs. Some employers and their industry associations would begin to talk about the need to seriously consider individual health insurance and thus withdraw altogether from financing health benefits for employees.

Status of Managed Care

Without being able to implement the traditional combination of a primary care gatekeeper and capitation of physicians (including specialists), managed care plans would continue to merge in order to increase their marketplace clout and reduce their costs. Some HMOs would back away from their practice of working with larger medical groups (primarily IPAs) and contract with smaller medical groups and even an occasional high-quality, cost-effective solo practitioner.

Health plans would aggressively invest in IT to monitor the quality and cost-effectiveness of individual physicians, medical groups, and hospitals and to stay ahead of the adoption of IT by providers. These advanced information systems would increase health plans' ability to tailor disease management programs to individual subscribers.

Managed care firms would find it necessary to develop new products in order to further diversify their product offerings. For the first time in the past two decades, there would be increasing interest on the part of consumers to self-insure against minor illnesses to make sure they have adequate coverage for major (catastrophic) needs, including access to new drugs and advanced medical procedures and devices.

Regarding the health insurance industry's ability to develop new products, Richard Huber, former chairman, CEO, and president of Aetna, said, "I can cover anything. I can write a policy that covers every conceivable experimental procedure, any number of in vitro fertilizations, and even hair transplants, as long as somebody pays for it. We don't make those (coverage) judgments. We can price it out, and if some payer, typically an employer, says, 'I want that for my employees,' terrific. I'll throw in Viagra, too. Whatever the buyer of the product wants, we can produce. Unfortunately we haven't done a very good job of making that clear" ("The Future of Health Care," 1999, p. 46). We believe that what Huber described would come to pass in this scenario. Consumers, including those on Medicare, would increasingly purchase insurance guaranteeing them access to medical technology and new drugs.

Role of Consumers

Already high consumer expectations for quality and service would continue to grow under the technology-dominant scenario. Everything we can learn from observing consumer behavior in other economic sectors affected by technological change points in this direction. And with consumers paying a bigger share of their own health care costs and insisting on more choice, we would expect dramatic change in terms of expectations from health care providers.

On a similar note the Institute for the Future says, "Both new consumers and, in fact, almost all health care consumers, want to be more involved in their health care than before. These consumers would exert their desire for involvement in two ways: by playing a much more active role in their own treatment decisions and by managing and providing their own care" (Institute for the Future, 1999, p. 4). The institute also states, "To the extent that their benefit designs allow it, people will feel much freer to switch away from plans and providers that don't meet their expectations for coverage, choice, speed, customer service, convenience, and information" (p. 4). In scenario 3 we expect to see this forecast begin to play out.

Health Care Market Growth

Under this scenario total health care spending would reach $1.9 trillion by 2005, or about $100 billion more than under the incremental-change scenario. Hospital revenues would increase, although these organizations would continue to lose market share. Physicians' share of health care spending would approximate 22 percent (compared with 20 percent under the incremental-change scenario). The share of the market garnered by drug companies would also be significantly higher than projected by most industry experts.

Internet and Clinical Information Systems

Spending on clinical IT would be higher than in the previous two scenarios. For the first time health care organizations would invest more than 2 to 3 percent of net revenues in IT. The admonitions of health care futurists to spend more on these kinds of systems and on research and development would finally be heeded. And of course the payoffs from these investments would begin to become evident by 2005.

A growing number of technology companies would develop new products for consumers. For example, many consumers would find it desirable to have their medical records stored electronically with for-profit firms.

Genetics, Drugs, and Medical Technology

As noted earlier, spending on drugs and medical technology by consumers, either through their health plans or out of pocket, would grow to unprecedented levels under this scenario. Genetic testing and gene therapy would become commonplace.

Spurred by the strong worldwide economy and their success in influencing consumers to insist on their brands, pharmaceutical companies would increase their spending on research and development and on direct-to-consumer advertising. Better information systems can be expected to reduce the incidence of errors in prescriptions, and patient compliance would improve.

A hot topic, and one of the most important public policy issues, would be the equity of denying new drugs to those who cannot pay the high costs. The gap between the haves and have-nots would widen. Many baby boomers would face the serious issue of whether or not to assist their aging parents in paying for promising new drugs.

Federal Policies

Under this scenario, with favorable economic conditions prevailing, the federal budget surplus would be large and growing. Thus concern over higher-than-anticipated Medicare spending would continue but would not be at the top of the public policy agenda. As Medicare expenditures exceeded the estimates developed in 1999, Congress and the president would face pressure to allocate money from budget surpluses to prop up Medicare. Public policy debate would focus on drug and high-tech company profits and incremental changes designed to reduce the number of the uninsured.

The Uninsured

Because of the strong economy and the success of incremental reforms like Medicare for those between the ages of fifty-five and sixty-four and CHIPS, the number of uninsured Americans would drop from around forty-five million in 2000 to around thirty to thirty-five million in 2005. This is still high but a substantial improvement over scenarios 1 and 2.

Consolidation

Health plans would be desperate to control technology-driven spending and improve profit margins; therefore consolidation to gain market clout and improve efficiency through economies of scale would be a high priority. The result: half a dozen national organizations, each with more than twenty million covered lives. The old saying that health care is a local business would begin to lose some of its relevance.

The financial pressures for hospitals and medical groups to consolidate would not be as great as in the first two scenarios. However, with health care becoming more national and international, many medical communities and smaller hospitals would be pressed to develop centers of excellence in order to compete. Smaller hospitals would lose some of their geographical advantage; it would become more difficult to hold patients from traditional service areas.

Scenario 3: Summary

In summary, under scenario 3 the impact of technology, especially the Internet and new drugs, would far exceed anything anticipated in 2000.

Scenario 4: Consumerism and Technology (Retail)

Scenario 4 (summarized in Exhibit 13.4) would combine scenario 3, technology dominant, with unprecedented growth in consumerism. As part of this scenario, employers would either get out of the health benefits business or implement defined contribution plans, vouchers, or MSAs. More radical payment models, such as the AMA individual-insurance proposal described in Chapter Twelve, would begin to be implemented.

Health plan executives would attend seminars on subjects such as how to achieve success in direct-to-consumer marketing. Physician seminars would include topics like meeting high and growing consumer expectations and dealing with consumer purchasing cooperatives. Because of their direct marketing success, pharmaceutical company executives would be in demand to speak at seminars on how to move consumers to buy your product.

Status of Managed Care

The most dramatic changes associated with this scenario would involve managed care. Health plans would increasingly market directly to consumers or consumer purchasing coalitions. Those health plans with prior experience in marketing Medicare risk products would be well positioned for this scenario.

Consumers would begin to form purchasing coalitions through churches, professional associations, labor unions, or other natural alliances. Some retail chains would offer health insurance plans to individuals. These purchasing cooperatives would be both national and local, with the national alliances offering consumers the added benefit of portability when they relocate or change jobs. Managed care plans would position themselves to deal with both purchasing alliances and individuals. However, some alliances would go around health plans and purchase health care directly from providers. As indicated in scenario 3, new types of health plans would develop to assist consumers in paying for drugs and advances in medical technology.

Role of Consumers

The consumer would reign supreme under this scenario. Health plan and provider choices available to consumers would be virtually

**Exhibit 13.4. Characteristics of Scenario 4:
Consumerism and Technology (Retail).**

Financial and Marketplace Factors	Characteristics
1. Prevalent payment system	1. Movement toward individual health insurance
2. Status of managed care	2. Managed care exists but in different forms, targeting different market segments (such as consumers and purchasing alliances rather than employers)
3. Economic conditions	3. Strong worldwide and U.S. economy
4. Role of consumers	4. Consumers are dominant; employers largely out of the picture
5. Health care market growth	5. $1.8 to $1.85 trillion by 2005
6. Internet and clinical information systems	6. Consumers demand state-of-the art communication and information systems
7. Genetics, drugs, and medical technology	7. Consumers insist on access to new drugs and technology and want new health plan alternatives that can guarantee access to technology
8. Federal policies	8. It takes a concerted federal policy and legislative effort to put individual health insurance model in place
9. The uninsured	9. Could decline to 20 to 25 million
10. Consolidation	10. Consolidation continues but for different reasons; focus on differentiation and providing value-added products and services

unlimited. To an unprecedented extent consumers would determine how much they want to spend and for what medical services. Because consumers would decide which health plans they want, the image of managed care would improve.

With the consumer in charge we would expect more interest in wellness, self-diagnosis, self-care, prevention, and CAM. Use of the Internet would be high, and a limited number of name brand Web sites would achieve acceptance and credibility. To an increasing extent physicians would be challenged by patients on their diagnosis and treatment plans.

Health Care Market Growth

The health care marketplace would grow to $1.85 trillion, a little below the technology-dominant scenario. We expect that if consumers spend more of their own money for health care, they will demand higher levels of service and be more sensitive to price differences and utilization might decline. In short, they would want more value added—quality, service, convenience, freedom of choice, personal relationships with physicians, affordability, information, and innovative approaches. We also expect hospitals and medical groups to operate more efficiently under this scenario, thus reducing administrative expenses and total health care spending.

Part of the growth in health care spending in this scenario would be attributable to international market development by U.S. physicians, hospitals, biomedical and drug companies, and producers of medical products. Using new approaches to telemedicine via the Internet and offering the most advanced medical technology and drugs in the world, a number of prestigious organizations would find ways to expand their services internationally. Health care would become one of America's biggest export industries.

People from various parts of the world—Mexico, South and Central America, Europe, and Asia—would have the disposable income to come to the United States for high-tech diagnostic and surgical procedures or would pay to have these services delivered in their home countries. The most prestigious health care organizations, like the Mayo Clinic, would have as much foreign business as they could handle.

Regarding the international development of health care, John Cochrane, editor of *Integrated Healthcare Report,* says:

> I think it will become a very small world, very soon. The Internet is exploding. There is no doubt, after seeing personally what is happening in Russia, that American health care organizations are missing the boat by not turning their attention to other countries. Baylor, for example, has an affiliation with the only clinic in Moscow; it is called the American Medical Center. This clinic is better equipped than any clinic in Moscow, and Western medicine is very distinctive from the herbal medicine practiced in large parts of Russia. Given the technology, there is no reason American medicine shouldn't become the standard of care worldwide [personal communication, Apr. 9, 1999].

A physician-administrator told us, "With the Internet and telemedicine, we are not constrained by how far we can reach out to patients. I mean, we can communicate instantaneously with patients in South America and the Middle East or anyplace else for that matter. There is an immense opportunity facing U.S. physicians and health care organizations. The issue is figuring out how to make a buck out of this and provide a service that is reasonable."

Internet and Clinical Information Systems

Scenario 4 would include all of the technological advances described in scenario 3. Under this scenario, it is difficult to believe (except in rural areas) that consumers would select physicians and hospitals that did not have the latest IT. Consumers would expect to be recognized when they check into a physician's office or hospital and would not stand for repetitive questions from support staff.

Genetics, Drugs, and Medical Technology

Consumers would be making their own choices in terms of the types of drug coverage they want to include in their health plan and how much to spend out of pocket on drugs. Drug company direct-to-consumer advertising would reach all-time highs. We expect consumers to be pleased with the results these new drugs can achieve, especially for the treatment of chronic illnesses, and the substitution of drug treatments for some surgeries.

It would become more common for consumers, particularly the elderly, who increasingly have access to sufficient financial resources, to either purchase supplemental insurance to cover drugs and technology or pay for more expensive medical procedures and products out of their own pockets. As a result, there would be heated controversies about the "unfairness" of a multitier health care system that, more and more, allows money to talk.

Federal Policies

HCFA would be faced with the issue of whether or not to incorporate the principles of individual insurance into Medicare and Medicaid. In scenario 4 the decision would be to move in this direction, initially through defined contributions, vouchers, and MSAs. (As noted in Chapter Twelve, HCFA is running a pilot program on MSAs.)

Of course, a primary federal policy issue related to increasing interest in individual-insurance models would be how to finance health care for the uninsured. The Heritage Foundation and AMA proposals recommend tax credits and deductions. However, this would be debated at length before a decision (and some progress in providing a payment source for some of the uninsured) was made.

With even partial implementation of the individual-insurance model, including universal coverage, physicians and hospitals would not be burdened with the excessive cost shifting typical in the year 2000 (discussed in Chapter Five). This would eliminate a major source of disequilibrium for the health care system, especially for hospitals.

Community Rating

The Heritage Foundation proposal for a consumer choice model calls for a return to community rating (with adjustments for age and sex but not for health status); the AMA proposal does not. Arguments in favor of community rating would include its simplification of the health care system, elimination of discriminatory practices against those with serious illnesses, and capability of dealing with the complexities of genetic testing.

On the last point, as it becomes feasible to identify individuals susceptible to certain genetically based diseases, a health insurance plan that charges higher premiums to those who are most likely to become ill simply would not work. Modified community rating of the type discussed in Chapter Two would eliminate many of the concerns about this issue.

In this scenario, however, we do not anticipate broad acceptance of community rating. Nonetheless, there would be increased discussion of the basic principles of health care insurance and debate over various alternatives, including a return to some form of community rating.

Consolidation

In this scenario there would be continuing pressure for physicians, medical groups, and hospitals to consolidate but for somewhat different reasons than in the other scenarios. For example, consumers would favor health care systems that already have a regional or national brand name or the potential to develop a reputation for quality and cost-effectiveness. Also, measuring and reporting clinical quality, which would be emphasized in this scenario, is more readily accomplished by larger groups of physicians. Consolidating to gain market clout with health plans would be less important.

Scenario 4: Summary

In this scenario organizations would focus on finding ways to differentiate themselves by virtue of the value-added characteristics they can offer consumers. There would be more emphasis on identifying consumer market segments and developing products and services for specific segments (such as seniors or women of childbearing age).

Conclusions

In our view none of the four scenarios described in this chapter is pie-in-the-sky or beyond the range of possibility. (As noted in Chapter Twelve, although there are many supporters of a single-payer system, we believe the probability of that model being implemented in the time frame considered in this book is negligible.) Table 13.1 compares key characteristics of each of the four scenarios.

Chapter Fourteen evaluates each of these scenarios in terms of which would represent the best health care system for the United States, the probabilities of each coming into being over the next five years, and whether these changes would constitute a fundamental market shift for health care.

Table 13.1. Summary of the Four Scenarios.

Financial and Marketplace Factors	Scenario 1: Incremental Change	Scenario 2: Constrained Resources	Scenario 3: Technology Dominant	Scenario 4: Consumerism and Technology (Retail)
1. Prevalent payment system	Employer-based managed care with some increase in defined contribution	Defined contribution more prevalent; private pay shrinks	Wide variety of payment systems; Medicare pays full cost; private pay explodes	Employers phasing out as payers; move toward vouchers, MSAs, and individual insurance models
2. Status of managed care	100 million covered lives (one-third of population)	120 million covered lives; shift to HMOs and away from PPOs	110 million covered lives; Medicare moves aggressively to managed care	110 million covered lives; emphasis changes to consumers
3. Economic conditions	Continuation of 1990s trends	Recession; drop in equity markets	Continuation of 1990s trends	Continuation of 1990s trends
4. Role of consumers	Continues to grow	More emphasis on self-care; less discretionary spending on health care	Continues to grow	Consumers take control
5. Health care market growth	$1.8 trillion	$1.6 trillion	$1.9 trillion	$1.85 trillion

Table 13.1. Summary of the Four Scenarios, *continued*

Financial and Marketplace Factors	Scenario 1: Incremental Change	Scenario 2: Constrained Resources	Scenario 3: Technology Dominant	Scenario 4: Consumerism and Technology (Retail)
6. Internet and clinical information systems	Continuing investment in IT; growing use of Internet	Investment in IT slows; Internet use increases	Increased investment in IT; explosion in use of Internet	Pressures to show benefits from investment in IT; Internet use high
7. Genetics, drugs, and medical technology	Continuing progress; many new drugs	Slowdown in drug sales	Boom in gene therapy; new drugs and medical technology; rapid adoption	More selectivity by consumers in purchase of drugs and use of technology
8. Federal policies	Slight relaxing of BBA; focus on compliance; strong antitrust enforcement	No relaxation of BBA; added emphasis on corporate compliance	Significant relaxation of BBA to improve payment to hospitals	Medicare shifts to vouchers and premium support
9. The uninsured	55 million (18%)	60 to 65 million (20+%)	30 to 35 million (10+%)	20 to 25 million (less than 10%)
10. Consolidation	Trends of late 1990s slow	Physician and hospital consolidation accelerates	Health plan consolidation accelerates	Physician and hospital consolidation continues

Learning from Analysis of the Four Scenarios

Although we don't know exactly how the future of health care will shape up, we can see the basic framework, and it involves a fundamental market shift toward consumerism and technology. Recognition of this shift has to drive our strategies, or else we will be left standing at the starting gate.

HEALTH SYSTEM CEO

This final chapter deals with three questions:

- Which of the four health care scenarios would be best for the country?
- Which of the scenarios is most likely to materialize? What are the probabilities associated with each scenario?
- Would scenarios 3 and 4 constitute a fundamental market shift for health care?

Which Scenario Is Best?

Our purpose here is to analyze each of the scenarios in terms of how well they satisfy ten criteria. Almost everyone has an opinion about what kind of health care system would be best. We are no different. We would like to see changes that would place the health care system on a sustainable financial basis and do a much better job of meeting consumer needs.

Seven Desirable Characteristics of a Sustainable Health Care System

In *The Crisis in Health Care: Costs, Choices and Strategies* (Coddington, Keen, Moore, and Clarke, 1990), we evaluated several scenarios for the future. Here are the seven criteria we used in evaluating various reform proposals:

1. Quality of care
2. Universal coverage
3. Cost stability
4. Choice of health plans and providers
5. Ease of administration
6. Financial stability
7. Cost shifting

We acknowledged in our previous book that there were many other factors that could have been included, but we suggested that these seven were the most important.

Additional Characteristics of a Sustainable Health Care System

Our thinking has changed somewhat since 1990. We believe that the seven criteria just defined are relevant as we enter the new millennium, especially financial stability and reduced cost shifting. However, we offer three more criteria that we believe have emerged as important:

1. *Innovation, product development, and service.* A health care system should enhance innovation, product development, and service. These are among the value-added characteristics most important to employers and consumers.
2. *Access to health care regardless of location.* The ideal system would ensure access to health care for residents of rural, inner-city, and other underserved areas.
3. *Coordinated system of care.* The best system would help to build a coordinated health care system that spans the continuum of care and offers meaningful disease management programs for chronic illnesses.

The paragraphs that follow describe each of the criteria used in our analysis of the four scenarios.

Criterion 1: Improves Quality of Care

This could be thought of as reducing clinical variation. We also consider the development and application of clinical guidelines, medical practice improvement initiatives, the continued development and use of clinical IT, and measuring clinical outcomes to be part of this criterion. All of these factors were discussed in Chapter Eight.

The unexplained large variations in medical practice in different communities with the same demographic characteristics are a continuing embarrassment to medicine. Dr. John Wennberg and his colleagues at Dartmouth have been documenting these variations for more than two decades. The variations do not appear to be getting any smaller.

Criterion 2: Provides Universal Coverage

As the failed Clinton reform efforts demonstrated, it is easier to agree on the desirability of providing universal coverage than to find ways to pay for it. We continue to believe that universal coverage is an essential characteristic of a desirable health care system, primarily because it would make the system work better. It would, for example, reduce the financial disparities between those who pay the full price of health care and those who receive medical services but pay little or nothing.

We believe that universal coverage could be made available to the uninsured at a much lower cost than the $100-plus billion estimate circulated at the time of the debate over the Clinton proposal. As we discussed earlier, the uninsured have access to the health care system but often use the system inappropriately (for example, through visits to hospital emergency rooms and inadequate use of primary care services). A system that provides timely access to primary care services would not be as expensive as the estimates widely quoted in 1993 and would be far superior in terms of quality of care for the uninsured.

Criterion 3: Brings Cost Predictability and Stability

For years payers have been asking for stability and predictability in their health care costs. Being able to predict health care costs at least a year in advance remains an elusive goal, but it is no less important than in the past for employers, HCFA, and states concerned about funding their share of Medicaid.

Health plans have attempted to make their costs more predictable by shifting the risk to providers through capitated arrangements. However, although capitation works well in some areas (such as California, Washington, and Arizona), it does not work in many other parts of the country, especially the more sparsely populated states.

There are other interesting approaches for bringing predictability and stability to costs. The BHCAG approach in the Twin Cities—similar to vouchers—aligns financial incentives among consumers, employers, and care systems.

Criterion 4: Offers Broader Choice of Health Plans and Providers

The desire on the part of consumers for more choice has come on strong over the past five years. Perhaps the value consumers attached to choice never left, and we just thought it had. In any event an increasing number of consumers want to be able to choose their own health plan, physicians, and hospitals. Employers have been responding by offering plans with increased freedom of choice. Consumers' desire for choice is in conflict with reducing the annual rate of increase in health care costs. This is one of the key issues, and dilemmas, facing health care in the next century.

Criterion 5: Improves Administration and Cuts Overhead

The U.S. health care system is tremendously complex and expensive to manage and administer. There are different estimates of the amount of overhead in the system, and most fall between 25 and 30 percent of total health care costs. This compares with less than 10 percent in Canada and a paltry 2 percent for Medicare. The high overhead of the U.S. health care system is one of the arguments advanced for a single-payer system. (Administrative expenses and their impact on overall health care costs were discussed in Chapter Four.)

A goal for any alternative health care scenario should be system simplification and reduced overhead. More of the available funds should go into medical care, prevention, clinical information systems, and research and development.

Criterion 6: Bolsters Financial Stability

Financial stability, or the lack of it, has become one of the most troublesome issues facing health care. A major part of this relates to increased costs and the prospects for acceleration of cost increases in the future (see Chapter Four). Financial instability is prevalent on both the payer and provider sides.

As discussed in Chapter Eleven, it is far from clear how the United States is going to pay for Medicare in the future; none of the alternatives are attractive. At the same time physicians and hospitals are uncertain about how they will be reimbursed and whether payment will be adequate to support existing service levels. Under the first two scenarios, incremental change and constrained resources, reimbursement levels will probably not be adequate. Present conditions create an environment of uncertainty in health care that is not conducive to rational strategic planning and decision making.

Criterion 7: Reduces Cost Shifting

Our position on the damaging nature of cost shifting on the scale it occurs in health care was discussed in Chapter Five. Any scenario for the U.S. health care system that does not come to grips with this issue should not receive a high rating.

By definition, if cost shifting is to be reduced, weaker payers have to be propped up. This refers primarily to the uninsured and Medicaid. Although Medicare was an adequate payer over most of the 1990s, there is substantial concern about the impact of the BBA on Medicare's future payment rates. Will Medicare payment continue to cover both direct and indirect expenses or only marginal costs?

Criterion 8: Enhances Innovation, Product Development, and Service

Some would argue that the proliferation of medical technology and new drugs is the biggest problem we face. However, it is unlikely that consumers would agree. From all evidence it appears consumers are 100 percent behind the new drugs and advanced medical technologies and want more.

We believe the health care system of the future should encourage continuing research and development in genetics, pharmaceuticals, advanced medical technology, and clinical IT. It is unlikely that this investment will lower costs; on the contrary, enhancing innovation and product development will add to health care costs. But to do otherwise would be inconsistent with the medical ethic and what we believe Americans expect from their health care system.

We anticipate major improvements in health care's service levels in the new millennium. In other words, we expect many in health care to work hard to make their organizations more user friendly. Although some would argue service quality and ease of system use have increased, we believe the potential for further enhancements is almost unlimited.

Criterion 9: Ensures Access to Health Care Services Regardless of Where Individuals Live

Why is this important? We are concerned that the general direction health care appears to be headed (for example, more emphasis on investor-owned managed care plans) may work against people living in rural and inner-city areas. These areas are not usually attractive health care markets, and the residents often do not have the income to pay for more than basic services.

The book *Managed Care in the Inner City* (Andrulis and Carrier, 1999, pp. x–xi) offers the following insights regarding the possible future directions of managed care:

> Both threat and opportunity lie ahead for inner-city residents in the evolving scenario of managed care in its various forms. The

threat is that individuals who are working poor or low income, who historically have found quality health care difficult to obtain, could be alienated further from the health care system of middle-class America. The great opportunity is that managed care's success in the inner city could bring about a major break from the past fragmented, patchwork way of getting health care, replacing it with a substantially more far-reaching system of care for these communities. No clear direction has emerged to date.

Market-driven health care is often not attracted to people living in small and unattractive markets. We saw evidence of this in the late 1990s when health plans withdrew their Medicare risk products from dozens of rural counties where average adjusted per capita costs were low and where the elderly population had many health care needs. Health care scenarios that show promise for alleviating some of these concerns should receive preferential consideration in evaluating the scenarios of the future.

Criterion 10: Encourages Development of a Coordinated System of Care, Especially for Chronically Ill Patients

Nancy Whitelaw and Gail Warden of the Henry Ford Health System in Michigan believe that there will be little improvement in how delivery systems provide care or in the outcomes of care until HCFA and other payers agree on a vision of how health care should be organized: "Without such a vision . . . it is difficult to evaluate various payment models. This vision should begin with commitments to a coordinated health care system that spans the continuum of care and to proactive, longitudinal chronic disease management" (Whitelaw and Warden, 1999, p. 133).

We agree with Whitelaw and Warden. In our research into integrated health care systems and in community health care needs assessments, we have seen how fee-for-service payment and the typical adversarial relationship between health plans and providers lead to fragmentation rather than coordination. Those health care scenarios that include more organized and coordinated ways of treating patients who are elderly or who have chronic diseases should be rated favorably.

Evaluation of the Four Scenarios

Table 14.1 compares each of the four scenarios against the ten criteria, using a rating system of three stars:

    * Does not satisfy the criterion
  ** Partially satisfies the criterion
*** Fully satisfies the criterion

Our purpose in this evaluation is to assess how well each scenario satisfies what we believe to be the characteristics of a desirable health care system for this country.

Scenario 1

Scenario 1, incremental change, does not score well. It is obvious from Table 14.1 that scenario 1 does not meet the requirements for an economically viable and sustainable health care system for the future. Given managed care's history of poor relationships with consumers and physicians, HMOs in particular face a steep uphill battle to reestablish their credibility. The problem will not be solved until managed care creates arrangements that can win the loyalty, commitment, and responsible participation of physicians and consumers. In our view this probably will not happen other than in scenario 4.

Scenario 2

Scenario 2 would be unpleasant for providers, health plans, and consumers. The constrained-resources scenario does best in contributing to cost stability. Other than this one attribute, it does not have much to commend it. Nevertheless, it has to be taken as a serious possibility in a five-year time frame.

Scenario 3

Scenario 3, technology dominant, fully satisfies one of the criteria—innovation and enhanced service—and partially meets three others. As we discuss shortly, we believe this is the most likely scenario.

Table 14.1. Evaluation of the Four Scenarios.

Financial and Marketplace Factors	Scenario 1: Incremental Change	Scenario 2: Constrained Resources	Scenario 3: Technology Dominant	Scenario 4: Consumerism and Technology (Retail)
1. Quality of care	**	*	**	***
2. Universal coverage	*	*	*	**
3. Cost stability	*	**	*	**
4. Broader choice	**	*	**	**
5. Ease of administration	*	*	*	**
6. Financial stability	*	*	*	**
7. Cost shifting	*	*	*	**
8. Innovation, improved service	**	*	***	***
9. Rural and inner-city access	*	*	*	**
10. Coordination of care	*	*	**	**

*Does not satisfy the criterion.
**Partially satisfies the criterion.
***Fully satisfies the criterion.

Scenario 4

Scenario 4, consumerism and technology (retail), rates the high-est. This scenario fully satisfies two of the criteria and partially satisfies the eight others. If this scenario went as far as full im-plementation of the individual-insurance model, it would fully sat-isfy two additional criteria—universal coverage and broader choice.

The Probabilities

Although our rating of the four scenarios may be interesting from a policy perspective, what will the health care marketplace of the future look like? This question is more politically realistic than our previous efforts to objectively rank the four scenarios.

We believe that scenario 3 has the highest probability of pre-dominating in 2005. Incremental change is unlikely to prevail; we assign it a 10 percent probability. We believe there is a 20 percent chance of scenario 2 prevailing in the first five years of the new mil-lennium. Scenario 4 is the most radical of any of the scenarios and would require significant government action in order to be fully implemented. We therefore believe this scenario has a 20 percent chance of being dominant. Our estimates of probabilities are sum-marized in Figure 14.1.

Considering the results of our analysis of which scenario would be most in the public interest, are we being cynical in our assign-ment of these probabilities? No. There is tremendous inertia and many vested interests in the U.S. health care system. There does not appear to be a national consensus or compelling grassroots support for some of the more radical parts of scenario 4, includ-ing full implementation of the individual-insurance model. (Of course, this could change if escalating health care costs and poor earnings cause an increasing number of midsize and large employ-ers to drop their health benefits.)

Furthermore, if economic conditions remain strong and cor-porate earnings are consistently high, we do not see much evi-dence that employers and labor unions are anxious to back away from their commitment to provide health benefits. We doubt

**Figure 14.1. Authors' Estimates of Probability
of Each Scenario Dominating in 2005.**

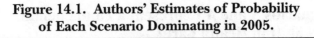

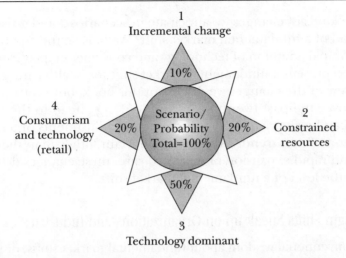

that most consumers would conclude that they would be just as well off with the individual-insurance proposal—more take-home pay to compensate for the loss of their health care insurance benefit. This is disappointing because we believe the AMA proposal for replacing employer-based coverage with individual insurance and other proposals for this model have much to commend them.

Based on what we have seen to date, we believe that the individual-insurance model deserves serious consideration. Both the AMA and the Heritage Foundation proposals have many worthwhile features, including the provision of universal coverage. Either would represent a vast improvement over the present fragmented employer-based system.

The BHCAG model used in the Twin Cities appears to have many positive attributes; perhaps it will catch on. It works reasonably well in a large metropolitan area where there is fierce competition among health care providers. But would it work for Medicare, and could it be successful in more rural areas? It would be useful to experiment with the BHCAG approach on a segment of the Medicare population.

Do Scenarios 3 and 4 Represent a Fundamental Market Shift in Health Care?

Do the kinds of changes we anticipate in scenarios 3 and 4 rise to the level of a fundamental market shift? We believe the combination of rapid adoption of technology and consumer empowerment would represent a fundamental market shift for health care.

Many of the changes we discuss in this book, both retrospectively over the past twenty years and looking ahead to the year 2005, can be characterized as incremental adjustments or a continuation of past trends. Although important, other than the advent and rapid expansion of managed care, these changes do not rise to the level of a fundamental market shift.

Paradigm Shifts Sneak up on Organizations and Industries

The conventional wisdom about fundamental market shifts, or paradigm shifts, is that those who are inside an industry do not drive these changes and often do not recognize them until after they have occurred. In other words, fundamental market shifts typically originate externally and from unlikely sources, often to the complete surprise of insiders. Examples are the development of the affordable automobile and the road building that eventually derailed passenger train travel, and the Three Mile Island power plant accident and the subsequent limitations on growth of the nuclear power industry.

Old Strategies Will Not Work

Many of the traditional ways of achieving success in any industry, including health care, will not work in the future. Kim Clark, dean of Harvard Business School, offers these observations:

> The other thing that is going to have profound consequences for the way business operates and the economy functions is the massive shift of power away from sellers to buyers—buyers in the consumer world, buyers in the business world. Buyers now have enormous power that they didn't have before. *So anybody who has made a business out of differentiating themselves on the basis of an information*

monopoly, or a locational advantage, may see their business disappear because this technology ruthlessly attacks those kinds of monopoly positions. That doesn't mean you won't be able to create differentiated advantage or margins, but they will have to be based on real value—some service, some technology, some concept you offer that is a superior value to those buyers—not just information. It hasn't all happened yet, but it is moving that way ["The Wired Society," 1999, p. 47, emphasis added].

When Clark talks about locational advantage and an information monopoly, it sounds like he is referring to health care. His comments combine two of the central themes of this book—the shift of power to buyers (primarily consumers) and away from sellers and the growth in technology.

Possible Drivers of a Fundamental Market Shift in Health Care

What could drive health care toward a fundamental shift in the next five years? We believe there are two critically important drivers and a third factor that should be considered.

- *Dramatically increased use of the Internet, new clinical IT, revolutionary new drugs, and an explosion in medical technology.* We have already seen evidence of the impact of new technology (such as laparoscopic surgery and laser eye surgery) and improved drugs. Although it has taken many years to realize benefits, the continuing high levels of investment in IT may begin influencing health care in significant ways by 2005. The more intensive use of much-improved and faster Internet services are bound to have tremendous impacts in terms of the way consumers interact with the health care system and the way physicians and other providers do business. Expansion of the U.S. health care system internationally would be facilitated by the Internet, telemedicine, new drugs, and advances in medical technology. This would be similar to the conditions we described in scenario 4.
- *Implementation of the individual-insurance model.* From a consumer perspective this would dramatically alter expectations for price and service improvements. Employers would be

shifting out of the health benefits business. The marketing efforts of health plans would be turned upside down. The implementation of something akin to the AMA or Heritage Foundation individual-insurance models would usher in a new era for health plans, physicians, hospitals, and consumers.

- *Failure to come to grips with the need to reduce the number of non-payers.* This could cause the employer-based system to begin to disintegrate. The uninsured and those on Medicaid would become more numerous, and those capable of paying full costs for health care services would shrink in number. We sometimes say this is analogous to the death spiral in indemnity insurance. The burden of paying for the uninsured and those receiving deep discounts (such as those on Medicaid) would overpower the base of employers and individuals that have been paying full cost or more.

We believe the impact of all aspects of technology (the Internet, IT, genetic research, new drugs, advances in medical technology) has the potential to radically change the U.S. health care system. Furthermore, the full power of the consumer has yet to be unleashed on health care. If these two forces join, as they would in scenario 4, the impact could be profound. Figure 14.2 shows the forces coming together to affect health care.

Conclusions

Is the health care glass half empty or half full? If we are talking about scenario 1, it is definitely half empty, with the water level dropping. However, the strong trend of consumers taking more control over their own health care leads us to believe that the glass is half full and the water level is rising.

We are concerned over the possible impact of an economic downturn and all that would be associated with such an adverse situation. Poor economic conditions, though, could force painful changes on the health care system (such as employers aggressively seeking ways to either eliminate health benefits for employees or reduce their costs) and set the stage for something more closely resembling the individual-insurance model. So even if this were to happen, we view it as having the potential to be a glass half full.

Figure 14.2. Strategic Inflection Point.

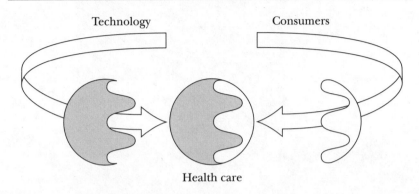

Either scenario 3 or 4 would be exciting for many in health care and could constitute a fundamental market shift. We have assigned scenario 3 the highest probability of predominating in the first five years of the twenty-first century. At the same time, since technology is one of the major drivers of health care costs, we are concerned about the effects this scenario could have on building a cost-effective health care system for the long term.

One of our objectives in writing this book was to assess past trends and current indicators in order to offer reasonable forecasts, or scenarios, of the health care system of the future. Our hope is that this analysis will stimulate the thinking of those who are concerned about health care in the United States and that the more positive health care futures will have a chance to develop. This is no time for a laissez-faire approach.

References

American Association for World Health. *Resource Booklet.* Washington, D.C.: American Association for World Health, 1999.

American Hospital Association. *AHA Hospital Statistics, 1993.* Chicago: American Hospital Association, 1993.

American Hospital Association. *AHA Hospital Statistics, 1996–97.* Chicago: American Hospital Association, 1996.

American Hospital Association. *The AHA Guide, 1998–1999 Edition.* Chicago: American Hospital Association, 1998.

American Medical Association. *Medical Group Practices in the U.S.: A Survey of Practice Characteristics.* (1993 ed.) Chicago: American Medical Association, 1993.

American Medical Association. *Empowering Our Patients: Individually Selected, Purchased and Owned Health Insurance Coverage.* Council on Medical Service Report, no. 9. Chicago: American Medical Association, 1998.

American Medical Association. *Medical Group Practices in the U.S.: A Survey of Practice Characteristics.* (1999 ed.) Chicago: American Medical Association, 1999a.

American Medical Association. *Rethinking Health Insurance.* Chicago: American Medical Association, 1999b.

Anderson, G. F. "In Search of Value: An International Comparison of Cost, Access, and Outcomes." *Health Affairs,* Nov.–Dec. 1997, pp. 163–171.

Andrulis, D. P., and Carrier, B. *Managed Care in the Inner City: The Uncertain Promise for Providers, Plans, and Communities.* San Francisco: Jossey-Bass, 1999.

Armey, D., and Stark, P. "Medical Coverage for All." *Washington Post,* June 18, 1999.

Arnett, G. M. *Empowering Health Care Consumers Through Tax Reform.* Ann Arbor: University of Michigan Press, 1999.

Astin, J. A. "Why Patients Use Alternative Medicine." *Journal of the American Medical Association,* 1998, *279,* 1548–1553.

Battistella, R., and Burchfield, D. "Defined Contribution: It's Inevitable." *Business and Health*, Nov. 1998, pp. 24–26.

Begley, S. "Screening for Genes: Matching Medications to Your Genetic Heritage." *Newsweek*, Feb. 8, 1999, p. 66.

Bellandi, D. "Consumers First." *Modern Healthcare*, Jan. 26, 1998, pp. 30–32.

Bellandi, D. "Sizing Up Systems." *Modern Healthcare*, Nov. 1, 1999, pp. 38–39.

Blumenthal, D. "Health Care Reform at the Close of the 20th Century." *New England Journal of Medicine*, 1999, *340*, 1916–1920.

Bodenheimer, T. "The American Health Care System: Physicians and the Changing Medical Marketplace." *New England Journal of Medicine*, 1999, *340*, 584–588.

Bodenheimer, T., Bernard, L., and Casalino, L. "Primary Care Physicians Should Be Coordinators, Not Gatekeepers." *Journal of the American Medical Association*, 1999, *280*, 2045–2049.

Brown, M. S. "Healthcare Information Seekers Aren't Typical Internet Users." *Medicine on the Net*, Feb. 1998, pp. 17–18.

Butler, S. M. "Have It Your Way: What the Heritage Foundation Health Plan Means for You." *Policy Review*, Fall 1993, pp. 54–59.

Butler, S. M., and Haislmaier, E. F. "The Consumer Choice Health Security Act." *Heritage Foundation Issue Bulletin*, Dec. 23, 1993, pp. 1–28.

Callahan, D. *False Hopes: Why America's Quest for Perfect Health Is a Recipe for Failure.* New York: Simon & Schuster, 1998.

Carrasquillo, O., Himmelstein, D. U., Woolhandler, S., and Bor, D. H. "A Reappraisal of Private Employers' Role in Providing Health Insurance." *New England Journal of Medicine*, 1999, *340*, 109–114.

Carrns, A. "Patients' Next Choice: Whether to Keep Files Stored on the Internet." *Wall Street Journal*, Aug. 16, 1999, p. B1.

"Chronic Care in America: The Health System That Isn't." *Advances*, 1996, *4*, 1, 9–10.

Clark, D. "Microsoft Brokers Healtheon-WebMD." *Wall Street Journal*, May 21, 1999, p. B6.

Cochrane, J. D. "Is Managed Care Going into a Stall?" *Integrated Healthcare Report*, Dec. 1998, pp. 1–13.

Cochrane, J. D. "Are Unions the Future of Medicine?" *Integrated Healthcare Report*, Feb. 1999a, pp. 1–12.

Cochrane, J. D. "Climbing Mount Everest: A Look at the Future of Healthcare." *Integrated Healthcare Report*, Mar. 1999b, pp. 14–15.

Coddington, D. C., Chapman, C. R., and Pokoski, K. M. *Making Integrated Health Care Work: Case Studies.* Englewood, Colo.: Center for Research in Ambulatory Health Care Administration, 1996.

Coddington, D. C., Keen, D. J., Moore, K. D., and Clarke, R. L. *The Crisis in Health Care: Costs, Choices, and Strategies.* San Francisco: Jossey-Bass, 1990.

Coddington, D. C., Moore, K. D., and Clarke, R. L. *Capitalizing Medical Groups: Positioning Physicians for the Future.* New York: McGraw-Hill, 1998.

Collins, F. S. "Shattuck Lecture: Medical and Societal Consequences of the Human Genome Project." *New England Journal of Medicine,* 1999, *341,* 28–37.

Conklin, M., "Quality Assurance: Kaiser's Regional President Makes HMO's Approach to Care a Priority." *Denver Rocky Mountain News,* Apr. 25, 1999, p. G4.

Cowley, G. "Beating the Back Ache." *Newsweek,* Mar. 15, 1999, p. 64.

"A Cyber Revolt in Health Care." *Business Week,* Oct. 19, 1998, pp. 154–156.

Dartmouth Medical School. *The Dartmouth Atlas of Health Care.* Chicago: American Hospital Publishing, 1996.

Deets, H. "Let the Countdown Begin to a Long, Healthy Life." *AARP Bulletin,* Jan. 1999, p. 28.

Dickey, N. W., and McMenamin, P. "Putting Power into Patient Choice." *New England Journal of Medicine,* 1999, *341,* 1305–1308.

Egger, E. "Drugs: Budget Busters or Cost Cutters in Future Health Care?" *Health Care Strategic Management,* Mar. 1999, pp. 1, 22–23.

Emanuel, E. J., and Emanuel, L. L. "The Economics of Dying: The Illusion of Cost Savings at the End of Life." *New England Journal of Medicine,* 1994, *330,* 540–544.

"Employer-Sponsored Health Plans." *Digest of Managed Health Care,* May 1998, pp. 2–4.

Enthoven, A. "The California Managed Health Care Improvement Task Force and the Future of HMOs." Presentation packet, Colorado Healthcare Strategy and Management meeting, Denver, May 27, 1998.

Eubanks, S., and Schauer, P. R. "Laparoscopic Surgery." In D. C. Sabiston Jr. (ed.), *Textbook of Surgery: The Biological Basis of Modern Surgical Practice.* (15th ed.) Philadelphia: Saunders, 1996.

Fifer, W. "A Doctor Looks at Alternative Care." *Will Fifer's Letters from Minneapolis,* May 1999, pp. 1–4.

Friedman, E. "Stop Me Before I Kill Again." *Healthcare Forum Journal,* Nov.–Dec. 1998, pp. 8, 10–12.

Fuchs, V. R. "Health Care for the Elderly: How Much? Who Will Pay for It?" *Health Affairs,* Jan.–Feb. 1999, pp. 11–21.

"The Future of Health Care: A *Harvard Magazine* Roundtable." *Harvard Magazine,* Mar.–Apr. 1999, pp. 43–51, 98–99.

Gates, B. *Business @ the Speed of Thought.* New York: Warner Books, 1999.

Gates, J. Presentation at the Healthcare in Transition: Physicians and Health Plans at the Crossroads conference, Denver, Apr. 9, 1999.

Gavora, C. J. "Back to the Drawing Board: Why Tax Reform Is the Key to Health Care Reform." *Heritage Foundation Backgrounder,* June 17, 1992, pp. 1–15.

Gawande, A. A., and others. "Does Dissatisfaction with Health Plans Stem from Having No Choices?" *Health Affairs,* Sept.–Oct. 1998, pp. 184–194.

Gemignani, J. "What's Holding Back MSAs?" *Business and Health,* Nov. 1997, pp. 34–39.

Gentry, C. "New England: So, What Is Anthem Doing in the Region—and Why?" *Wall Street Journal,* Feb. 17, 1999a [on-line].

Gentry, C. "UnitedHealth Move on Reviews Is Seen as Industry Watershed." *Wall Street Journal,* Nov. 10, 1999b, p. B6.

Gianelli, D. "Stem Cell Research Focus of Ethical Dilemma." *American Medical News,* Dec. 21, 1998, pp. 1, 34.

Gilbert, S. "New Treatment Shrinks Fibroids." *Denver Post,* Apr. 6, 1999, p. A12.

Gilkey, R. W. *The 21st Century Health Care Leader.* San Francisco: Jossey-Bass, 1999.

Ginzberg, E. "The Uncertain Future of Managed Care." *New England Journal of Medicine,* 1999, *340,* 144–146.

Golden, F. "Good Eggs, Bad Eggs." *Time,* Jan. 11, 1999a, pp. 56–59.

Golden, F. "Patrick Steptoe and Robert Edwards: Brave New Baby Doctors." *Time,* Mar. 29, 1999b, p. 178.

"Goldilocks or Gridlock?" *The Economist,* June 19, 1999, p. 17.

Goldsmith, J. "Operation Restore Human Values." *Hospitals and Health Networks,* July 5, 1998a, pp. 74, 76.

Goldsmith, J. "Three Predictable Crises in the Health System and What to Do About Them." *Healthcare Forum Journal,* Nov.–Dec. 1998b, pp. 42–46.

Gorman, C. "Drugs by Design." *Time,* Jan. 11, 1999, pp. 79–83.

Gorner, P. "Q&A with Arnold S. Relman, M.D." *Chicago Tribune,* Nov. 30, 1998.

Grumbach, K., and Fry, J. "Managing Primary Care in the United States and in the United Kingdom." *New England Journal of Medicine,* 1993, *228,* 940–945.

Hallam, K. "HHS: No Quick Fix for Hospital Woes." *Modern Healthcare,* May 31, 1999, p. 25.

Hays, P. "Healthcare Paradoxes in the New Millennium." *Integrated Healthcare Report,* Sept. 1998, pp. 1–5.

HCIA. *The Guide to the Managed Care Industry.* Baltimore: HCIA, 1998.

Health Care Financing Administration. "Medicare Enrollment Trends, 1966–1998." [www.hcfa.gov/stats/enrltrnd.htm]. June 30, 1999.

"Health Care: It's Better If You're White." *The Economist,* Feb. 27, 1999, p. 28.

Hofgard, M. W., and Zipin, M. L. "Complementary and Alternative Medicine: A Business Opportunity?" *MGM Journal,* May–June 1999, pp. 16–27.

Howgill, M.W.C. "Health Care Consumerism, the Information Explosion, and Branding: Why 'Tis Better to Be the Cowboy Than the Cow." *Managed Care Quarterly,* Fall 1998, pp. 33–43.

Hubler, E. "Doctors Begin New ER: Electronic Research." *Denver Post,* Apr. 4, 1999, p. J4.

Iglehart, J. K. "The American Health Care System—Expenditures." *New England Journal of Medicine,* 1999a, *340,* 70–76.

Iglehart, J. K. "The American Health Care System—Medicare." *New England Journal of Medicine,* 1999b, *340,* 327–332.

Iglehart, J. K. "Support for Academic Medical Centers: Revisiting the 1997 Balanced Budget Act." *New England Journal of Medicine,* 1999c, *340,* 299–304.

Institute for the Future. "Executive Summary: 1998 Health Care Ten Year Forecast." [www.iftf.org]. Menlo Park, Calif.: Institute for the Future, 1997.

Institute for the Future. "Executive Summary: 'New' Health Care Consumer." [www.iftf.org]. May 1998.

Institute for the Future. "The Internet and the Future of Telehealth." White paper sponsored by the California Healthcare Foundation, Jan. 1999.

Intel Corp. "Internet Health Day," San Francisco, Oct. 27, 1998. Proceedings available on-line [www.intel.com].

InterStudy. *The InterStudy Competitive Edge, Part II: HMO Industry Report.* St. Paul, Minn.: InterStudy, 1997.

Jaroff, L. "Fixing the Genes." *Time,* Jan. 11, 1999, pp. 68–73.

Jeffrey, N. A. "Paper Chases of a Cancer Patient." *Wall Street Journal,* Mar. 1, 1999, pp. B1, B4.

Johnston, M. D. "'Patient-Dumping' Horrors Heard." *Denver Post,* Feb. 18, 1999, p. A4.

Kaiser Family Foundation. "The Uninsured and Their Access to Health Care." Fact sheet, July 16, 1999.

Kaiser Industries. "The Prescription for Health." In Kaiser Industries, *The Kaiser Story.* Oakland, Calif.: Kaiser Industries, 1984, pp. 55–59.

Kalamas, J., Pinkus, G., Wang, N., and Zino, R. "Payor or Preyer?" *McKinsey Quarterly,* 1999(1), 52–61.

Kelly, J. T. "'After the Chaos': Expected Benefits of Health Information Management." *Health Affairs*, Nov.–Dec. 1998, pp. 39–40.

Kirkwood, D. H. "Dispensers in Survey Take Satisfaction in Their Work, but Many Feel Unappreciated." *Hearing Journal*, Mar. 1999, pp. 19–32.

Kuttner, R. "Must Good HMOs Go Bad? The Commercialization of Prepaid Group Health Care." *New England Journal of Medicine*, 1998a, *338*, 1558–1563.

Kuttner, R. "Must Good HMOs Go Bad? The Search for Checks and Balances." *New England Journal of Medicine*, 1998b, *338*, 1635–1639.

Kuttner, R. "The American Health Care System: Employer-Sponsored Health Coverage." *New England Journal of Medicine*, 1999, *340*, 248–252.

Lagnado, L. "Drug Costs Can Leave Elderly a Grim Choice: Pills or Other Needs." *Wall Street Journal*, Nov. 17, 1998, pp. A1, A8.

Lagnado, L. "Hospital Mergers: Indications of Severe Trauma." *Wall Street Journal*, May 14, 1999, pp. B6, B7.

Langreth, R. "Drugs Based on Genes Enter Human Trials." *Wall Street Journal*, Mar. 26, 1999, pp. B1, B4.

Langreth, R., and Moore, S. D. "Gene Therapy, Touted as a Breakthrough, Bogs Down in Details." *Wall Street Journal*, Oct. 27, 1999, pp. A1, A6.

Langreth, R., Waldholz, M., and Moore, S. D. "Big Drug Firms Discuss Linking Up to Pursue Disease-Causing Genes." *Wall Street Journal*, Mar. 4, 1999, pp. A1, A6.

"Lawrence Predicts Real Changes in Healthcare Are Yet to Come." *Modern Healthcare*, Jan. 18, 1999, p. 40.

Lazarus, S. S. "Physicians' Use of Electronic Medical Records." *MGM Journal*, May–June 1999, pp. 1–13.

Lemonick, M. D. "On the Horizon." *Time*, Jan. 11, 1999, p. 89.

Lemonick, M. D., and Thompson, D. "Racing to Map Our DNA." *Time*, Jan. 11, 1999, pp. 44–50.

Lutz, S., and Gee, E. P. *Columbia/HCA: Healthcare on Overdrive*. New York: McGraw-Hill, 1998.

Maller, B. "Refractive Surgery: Is It Too Late to Get in the Game?" *Administrative Eyecare*, Winter 1999, pp. 49–51.

McGinley, L. "As Nursing Homes Say, 'No,' Hospitals Feel Pain." *Wall Street Journal*, May 26, 1999, pp. B1, B4.

McLaughlin, N. "Blame on You." *Modern Healthcare*, Feb. 8, 1999, p. 58.

McNeil, J. *Changes in Median Household Income, 1969 to 1996*. Current Population Reports, Special Studies, P23-196. Washington, D.C.: U.S. Department of Commerce, Bureau of the Census, 1998.

Medical Benefits, Apr. 15, 1998.

Medicare Payment Advisory Committee. *Report to the Congress: Medicare Payment Policy.* Washington, D.C.: Social Security Administration, Mar. 1999.

"Medicare Reform: Promises, Promises." *The Economist,* Mar. 27, 1999, pp. 29, 32.

Mettler, M. "Lessons Learned: The Empowered and Informed Healthcare Consumer." [www.healthwise.org]. 1999a.

Mettler, M. "The 21st Century Healthcare Consumer." [www.healthwise.org]. 1999b.

Mittman, R. "Forecasting the Pace of Change in Health Care." Institute for the Future [www.iftf.org], Jan. 21, 1999.

Moffit, R. E. "Why the Maryland Consumer Choice Health Plan Could Be a Model for Health Care Reform." *Heritage Foundation Backgrounder,* June 17, 1992.

Moore, P. "Physician Glut Numbers Exaggerated, Speaker Says." *Medical Group Management Update,* Aug. 15, 1999, p. 3.

"1999 Industry Outlook." *Healthcare Trends Report,* Jan. 1999, pp. 1–22.

O'Brien, C. F. "Movement and Function: Current Understanding and Care." *CNI Review,* Winter 1998–1999, pp. 3–8.

Pear, R. "Insurers Ask Government to Extend Health Plans." *New York Times,* May 23, 1999, p. Y16.

PricewaterhouseCoopers and Lutz, S. *Physician Group Management at the Crossroads.* New York: McGraw-Hill, 1999.

Quinn, J. B. "The Invisible Uninsured." *Newsweek,* Mar. 1, 1999, p. 49.

Rauber, C. "Can't Shake the Blues." *Modern Healthcare,* Mar. 22, 1999, p. 14.

Reese, S. "What's Next?" *Business and Health,* Jan. 1999, pp. 30–35.

Reinertsen, J. L. "Leading Clinical Quality Improvement: Political and Practical Milestones, Part 1." *Healthcare Forum Journal,* July–Aug. 1994, pp. 19–24.

Robinson, J. C. "The Future of Managed Care Organization." *Health Affairs,* Mar.–Apr. 1999, pp. 7–24.

Ross, J. R. "Healthy Ambition." *Harvard Business School Bulletin,* June 1999, p. 31.

Rundle, R. L. "The Outlook: Can Managed Care Manage Costs?" *Wall Street Journal,* Aug. 9, 1999, p. A1.

Sardegna, C. J. "How the Maryland Health Plan Is a Model for the Nation." Lecture no. 392, May 27, 1992.

Schwartz, W. B. *Life Without Disease: The Pursuit of Medical Utopia.* Berkeley: University of California Press, 1998.

Shalala, D. E., and Reinhardt, U. E. "Viewing the U.S. Health Care System from Within: Candid Talk from HHS." *Health Affairs,* May–June 1999, pp. 47–55.

Shearer, G. "Hidden from View: The Growing Burden of Health Care Costs." *Consumer Report,* Jan. 22, 1998.

Shinkman, R. "Premiums Rising for All Types of Plans." *Modern Healthcare,* Mar. 29, 1999, p. 66.

Shutan, B. "Health Cash Accounts Ride Cash Balance Coattails." *Employee Benefit News,* Aug. 1999, pp. 18–19.

Smith, S., and others. "The Next Ten Years of Health Spending: What Does the Future Hold?" *Health Affairs,* Sept.–Oct. 1998, pp. 128–140.

Soumerai, S. B., and Ross-Degnan, D. "Inadequate Prescription-Drug Coverage for Medicare Enrollees: A Call to Action." *New England Journal of Medicine,* 1999, *340,* 722–728.

Starr, P. *The Social Transformation of American Medicine.* New York: Basic Books, 1982.

Stevens, L. "Virtually There." *American Medical News,* Dec. 21, 1998, pp. 24–27.

Tanouye, E. "Drug Dependency: U.S. Has Developed an Expensive Habit; Now, How to Pay for It?" *Wall Street Journal,* Nov. 15, 1998.

Tikker, B. Presentation at the Crossroads conference, Healthcare in Transition: Physicians and Health Plans, Denver, Apr. 9, 1999.

"Uncovered Lives." *Modern Healthcare,* Mar. 15, 1999, p. 64.

U.S. Department of Commerce, Bureau of the Census. *Resident Population of the United States: Middle Series Projections, 1996–2000.* Washington, D.C.: U.S. Government Printing Office, 1996.

U.S. Department of Health and Human Services. *A Profile of Medicare: Chart Book.* Washington, D.C.: U.S. Government Printing Office, 1998.

U.S. Department of Health and Human Services. "Health in America Tied to Income and Education." *HHS News,* July 13, 1999, pp. 1–4.

VHA Inc. *Provider-Based Managed Care Networks—and Beyond.* Dallas: VHA Inc., 1996.

Vladeck, B. C. "Plenty of Nothing: A Report from the Medicare Commission." *New England Journal of Medicine,* 1999, *340,* 1503–1506.

Waldholz, M., and Tanouye, E. "Glaxo to Report It's Closing In on Genes Linked to 3 Diseases." *Wall Street Journal,* Oct. 19, 1999, pp. A1, A12.

Walker, T. "Seniors Dig Deep to Pay for Healthcare Coverage." *Managed Healthcare,* Apr. 1998, pp. 6, 9.

Weeks, W. B., Kofoed, L. L., Wallace, A. E., and Welch, H. G. "Directives and the Cost of Terminal Hospitalization." *Archives of Internal Medicine,* 1994, *154* (18), 2077–2083.

Welch, W. M., and Page, S. "Drug Benefit Newest Twist in Debate over Medicare." *USA Today,* Apr. 29, 1999, pp. A1–A2.

Whitelaw, N., and Warden, G. "Reexamining the Delivery System as Part of Medicare Reform." *Health Affairs,* Jan.–Feb. 1999, pp. 132–143.

Windhorst, C. "Alternative Medicine's Potent Attraction for Boomers and Seniors." *Healthcare Strategist,* Oct. 1998, pp. 7–8.

Winslow, R. "Elderly Need Preventive Care but Don't Get It." *Wall Street Journal,* Apr. 19, 1999a, pp. B1, B4.

Winslow, R. "Study Suggests Tool to Fight Heart Disease." *Wall Street Journal,* Apr. 6, 1999b, pp. B1, B4.

"The Wired Society: A *Harvard Magazine* Roundtable." *Harvard Magazine,* May–June 1999, pp. 42–53, 106–107.

Woolhandler, S., Himmelstein, D. U., and Lewontin, J. P. "Administrative Costs in U.S. Hospitals." *New England Journal of Medicine,* 1993, *329,* 400–403.

Index

Epigraph Credits

Preface: J. D. Cochrane, "Is Managed Care Going into a Stall?" *Integrated Health-care Report,* Dec. 1998, p. 3.

Part One: S. Lutz and E. P. Gee, *Columbia/HCA: Healthcare on Overdrive.* New York: McGraw-Hill, 1998, p. 5.

Chapter One: J. Goldsmith, "Operation Restore Human Values." *Hospitals and Health Networks,* July 5, 1998, p. 74.

Chapter Two: R. Kuttner, "Must Good HMOs Go Bad? The Commercialization of Prepaid Group Health Care." *New England Journal of Medicine,* 1998, *338,* 1558.

Chapter Four: J. Daniel Beckham, "The Obsolescence of Independent Practice," *Heath Forum Journal,* Mar.–Apr. 1999, p. 38.

Chapter Five: D. C. Coddington, D. J. Keen, K. D., Moore, and R. L. Clarke, *The Crisis in Health Care: Costs, Choices, and Strategies.* San Francisco: Jossey-Bass, 1990, p. 112.

Part Three: "Lawrence Predicts Real Changes in Healthcare Are Yet to Come," *Modern Healthcare,* Jan. 18, 1999, p. 40.

Chapter Six: Institute for the Future. "Executive Summary: 'New' Health Care Consumer" [www.iftf.org]. May 1998, p. 3.

Chapter Seven: M. Hassett and M. Rybarski, "Transforming and Repositioning Healthcare for the Boomers," *Healthcare Strategist,* Feb. 1999, p. 1.

Chapter Eight: "The Wired Society: A *Harvard Magazine* Roundtable," *Harvard Magazine,* May–June 1999, p. 44.

Chapter Nine: D. Callahan, *False Hopes: Why America's Quest for Perfect Health Is a Recipe for Failure.* New York: Simon & Schuster, 1998, p. 73. Reprinted with the permission of Simon & Schuster. Copyright © 1998 by Daniel Callahan.

Chapter Ten: J. Koster, personal interview, Mar. 12, 1999.

Chapter Twelve: R. Kuttner, "The American Health Care System: Employer-Sponsored Health Coverage." *New England Journal of Medicine,* 1999, *340,* 252.

Part Four: R. Kuttner, "Must Good HMOs Go Bad? The Search for Checks and Balances." *New England Journal of Medicine,* 1998b, *338,* 1638.

General Credits

Chapter Eight: List on p. 160 from "Physician's Use of Electronic Medical Records," by Stephen S. Lazarus, originally appeared in *Medical Group Management Journal* 46(3), May–June, 1999. Reprinted with permission from the Medical Group Management Association, 104 Inverness Terrace East, Englewood, Colorado 80112-5306; 303-799-1111. Copyright 1999.